Updates in Endoscopy

Edited by Somchai Amornyotin

Published in London, United Kingdom

Updates in Endoscopy
http://dx.doi.org/10.5772/intechopen.102227
Edited by Somchai Amornyotin

Contributors
Anabela Serranito, Lorenzo Capone, Bahadir Kartal, Mehmet Abdussamet Bozkurt, William B. Stetson, Katie Lutz, Kristen Reikersdorfer, Lubna Kamani

First published in London, United Kingdom, 2023 by IntechOpen
IntechOpen is the global imprint of INTECHOPEN LIMITED, registered in England and Wales, registration number: 11086078, 5 Princes Gate Court, London, SW7 2QJ, United Kingdom

British Library Cataloguing-in-Publication Data
A catalogue record for this book is available from the British Library

Additional hard and PDF copies can be obtained from orders@intechopen.com

Updates in Endoscopy
Edited by Somchai Amornyotin
p. cm.
Print ISBN 978-1-83769-982-7
Online ISBN 978-1-83768-200-3
eBook (PDF) ISBN 978-1-83768-201-0

Meet the editor

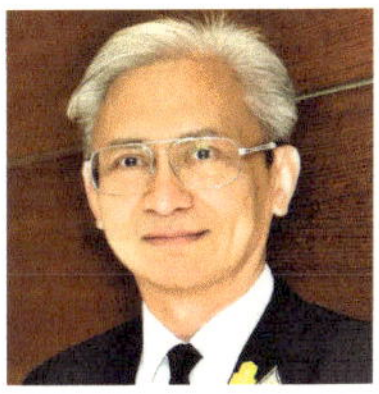

Dr. Somchai Amornyotin received his medical degree from the Faculty of Medicine at Siriraj Hospital, Mahidol University, Bangkok, Thailand in 1989. In 1996, he joined the Department of Anesthesiology at the same hospital and went on to become a professor in 2020. Dr. Amornyotin's research career began with his first scientific paper published in Thailand in 1999, and since then he has published over 80 research articles in both Thai and international medical journals. He is a member of various professional organizations such as the Royal College of Anesthesiologists of Thailand and the Gastroenterological Association of Thailand, and is also a reviewer and editor for numerous international journals.

Contents

Preface

The edited volume *Updates in Endoscopy* is a comprehensive collection of research chapters that highlights the latest advancements in the field of endoscopy. The book is edited by a group of experts in health sciences, and each chapter is written by a specialist in the field. While each chapter is self-contained, all are related to the book's overarching themes and objectives. This book is targeted at scholars and specialists in the field who seek to deepen their understanding of endoscopy and stay up to date with the latest developments.

Dr. Somchai Amornyotin
Faculty of Medicine,
Department of Anesthesiology,
Siriraj Hospital,
Mahidol University,
Salaya, Thailand

Chapter 1

Upper and Lower Gastrointestinal System Endoscopy Indications

Bahadir Kartal and Mehmet Abdussamet Bozkurt

Abstract

As endoscopic procedures have become widespread, they have largely replaced radiological methods in the diagnosis of gastrointestinal system diseases; because the accurate diagnosis rates of endoscopic procedures are very high compared to conventional radiological procedures. In addition, tissue and cell sample for histopathological studies It is also advantageous because it can be taken and some diseases can be treated endoscopically. Rigid endoscopes have been replaced by flexible endoscopes, making them widely used in both diagnosis and treatment. The increase in the use of endoscopy brings with it complications. Therefore, the indications for endoscopy should be clearly stated. Indications for endoscopic examination of the digestive system can be divided into three as diagnosis, follow-up and treatment.

Keywords: gastroscopy, colonoscopy, indication, gastrointestinal endoscopy

1. Introduction - Upper gastrointestinal system endoscopy indications

With the widespread use of flexible endoscopes, the indications for upper gastrointestinal endoscopy (Upper GI) have increased. Upper GI indications; It is divided into three as diagnostic, follow-up and therapeutic (**Table 1**).

2. Diagnostic upper GI

2.1 Dyspepsia

Upper GI should be performed in patients aged 50 years and older in the presence of new-onset dyspepsia. If under 50 years of age, medical treatment should be given. Endoscopy should be performed if the following alarm symptoms are present with dyspepsia.

Alarm symptoms:

- Persistent vomiting
- Progressive dysphagia
- Obstructive jaundice

Diagnostic	Follow-up	Therapeutic
Dyspepsia	Achalasia	Foreign body
GERD	Tylosis	Upper gastrointestinal bleeding
Upper gastrointestinal bleeding	PUD	Endoskopic resections
Dysphagia and odynophagia	Barrett's esophagus	Polypectomy
Vomiting	Polyps	Dilation and stent
Caustic injury	Intestinal metaplasia/ dysplasia	PEG/ PEJ
Iron deficiency anemia	Post – gastric surgery	Ablation
	Pernicious anemia	Achalasia
	FAP	Obesity
	HNPCC	
	History of upper respiratory and digestive tract cancer	

FAP: Familial Adenomatous Polyposis, HNPCC: Hereditary Nonpolyposis Colorectal Cancer, PEG: Percutaneous endoscopic gastrostomy, PEJ: Percutaneous endoscopic jejunostomy, GERD: Gastroesophageal reflux disease, PUD: Peptic ulcer disease.

Table 1.
Upper gastrointestinal system endoscopy indications.

- Dysphagia or odynophagia
- Involuntary loss of more than 3 kg in the last two months
- Palpable mass in the epigastrium or peripheral lymphadenopathy
- Upper gastrointestinal bleeding
- Iron deficiency anemia
- Family history of upper gastrointestinal malignancy

Upper GI is performed to diagnose Helicobacter pylori or evaluate response to treatment. Upper GI should be performed in patients with dyspeptic complaints who are taking empirical proton pump inhibitors if they do not respond to treatment [1, 2].

2.2 Gastroesophageal reflux disease

Gastroesophageal reflux disease can be diagnosed with typical (heartburn, regurgitation) symptoms and treated if uncomplicated. However, Upper GI should be performed in patients with alarm symptoms or who do not respond to treatment [3].

2.3 Upper gastrointestinal bleeding

If the patient has signs of bleeding from the upper gastrointestinal tract, such as hematemesis and/or melena, Upper GI should be performed [4].

2.4 Dysphagia and odynophagia

The first examination to be performed in patients with dysphagia and odynophagia is endoscopy. If there is progressive dysphagia against solid foods, rapid endoscopy should be planned [5].

2.5 Vomiting

Upper GI should be performed if patients have persistent (more than 48 hours) vomiting and the vomiting is thought to originate from the digestive system [1, 2].

2.6 Caustic injury

EGD is performed to determine the extent and severity of damage in patients taking corrosive substances [6].

2.7 Iron deficiency anemia

Patients over 50 years of age with iron deficiency anemia should also undergo colonoscopy with EGD. A duodenal biopsy is also necessary to investigate celiac disease in patients with iron deficiency anemia [7].

3. Follow-up upper GI

Upper GI is used in the follow-up of some benign, malignant and malignancy-risk diseases.

3.1 Achalasia

Since the onset of the disease, the risk of developing squamous cell cancer has increased. Upper GI should be performed in these patients every 3 years [8].

3.2 Tylosis

Tylosis is an autosomal dominant skin disease. Type A tylosis, which occurs at between the ages of 5 and 15 years and is associated with squamous cell carcinoma of the esophagus. Endoscopic brush cytology once a year and chromoendoscopy every 3 years should be planned at least 10 years before the age at which the diagnosis is usually made in the affected family member [9].

3.3 Peptic ulcer disease

In patients diagnosed with gastric ulcer by biopsy, a control endoscopy should be performed after 4–6 weeks of antisecretory therapy. In patients diagnosed with duodenal ulcer with Upper GI, if there are no symptoms after 4–6 weeks of treatment, there is no need to do endoskopy again [6].

3.4 Barrett's esophagus

In patients with Barrett's esophagus with no evidence of dysplasia on initial endoscopy, a repeat endoscopy should be performed within the next year. Annual endoscopy has been recommended for Barrett's esophagus with low- grade dysplasia [10]. Barret's patients with high- grade dysplasia should undergo Upper GI at frequent intervals (every 3 months) (4-quadrant jumbo biopsies) [11].

3.5 Gastric epithelial polyps

Fundic gland polyps have not been associated with an increased risk of cancer. But, hyperplastic polyps have a rare malignant potential. Adenomatous polyps have malignant potential and this risk correlates with size and older patient age. Biopsy or polypectomy is recommended when a polyp is encountered. Surveillance endoscopy should be planned 1 year after removal of adenomatous gastric polyps. If high-grade dysplasia or early gastric cancer is detected in the follow-up, the necessary treatment should be performed. If the results of this examination are negative, repeat surveillance endoscopy should be performed at 3 to 5 year intervals. No surveillance endoscopy is necessary after adequate sampling or removal of nondysplastic gastric polyps [12].

3.6 Gastric intestinal metaplasia and dysplasia

The risk of developing gastric cancer is 10 times higher in patients with intestinal metaplasia. If low grade dysplasia is detected in a patient with intestinal metaplasia, then surveillance Upper GI with a topographic mapping biopsy strategy should be performed every 3 months, at least for the first year. Surveillance should be suspended when 2 consecutive endoscopies show a negative result. Patients with high grade dysplasia should undergo gastrectomy or endoscopic resection [12].

3.7 Post - gastric surgery

There is insufficient evidence to support the need for routine endoscopic follow-up in patients who have undergone partial gastrectomy for peptic ulcer. In these patients, if there are symptoms, Upper GI should be performed. If surveillance is considered, it should be initiated after an interval of 15 to 20 years [13]. Preoperative Upper GI should be performed in patients scheduled for bariatric surgery [14].

3.8 Pernicious anemia and gastric carcinoid tumors

There are an increased risk of gastric cancer, as well as gastric carcinoid tumors, in patients with pernicious anemia. The benefits of surveillance in patients with pernicious anemia have not been shown. A single endoscopy should be considered to identify lesions (gastric cancer, carcinoid tumors) in patients with pernicious anemia. The follow-up of carcinoid tumors should be personalized according to the patient [15].

3.9 Familial adenomatous polyposis (FAP)

Fundic gland polyps are found in 88% of FAP patients [16]. Adenomatous polyps are found in the stomachs of individuals with FAP, with a prevalence ranging from 2–50% [17]. They are usually located in the antrum. Duodenal adenomas occur in

90% of patients with adult FAP [16]. Duodenal adenomas are usually formed in the duodenal papillae or in the periampullary region. Spigelman classification is used for duodenal polyposis classification [18]. The optimal timing of the first Upper GI of patients with FAP is unknown, but it can be performed around the time when the patient is being considered for colectomy, or at the beginning of the third decade of life. If adenoma is not detected, a re-examination should be performed after 5 years, as there may be adenomatous changes later in the course of the disease. If excision of the papillary adenoma has been complete, one approach is for follow-up endoscopy and multiple biopsies every 6 months for a minimum of 2 years, with endoscopy thereafter at 3-year intervals [12].

3.10 Hereditary nonpolyposis colorectal cancer (HNPCC)

Patients with HNPCC are at increased risk for the development of gastric and small-bowel cancer [19]. Upper GI follow-up is appropriate from the age of 30 [20].

3.11 History of upper respiratory tract cancer and upper digestive tract cancer

There are insufficient data to support routine endoscopic surveillance. A single Upper GI is recommended to identify esophageal cancer [21].

4. Therapeutic upper GI

4.1 Removal of foreign bodies

During the removal of a foreign body, an overtube provides some degree of protection of the airway. The overtube is also useful for protecting the mucosa when it is necessary to pass the endoscope several times to remove a foreign body. After removal of the foreign body, the endoscope should be reinserted in case of adverse events [22].

4.2 Upper gastrointestinal bleeding

In case of upper gastrointestinal bleeding, epınephrıne ınjectıon, sclerosants, tissue adhesive, thermal coagulatıon, hemospray, band ligation and hemoclıps can be performed by Upper GI [23].

4.3 Endoscopic resections

Endoskopic mucosal resection (EMR) is used to excise focal lesions of the mucosa. The lesions are most commonly located in the stomach. Endoscopic submucosal dissection (ESD) allows for en bloc excision of large mucosal lesions of the gastrointestinal tract [22, 23].

4.4 Polypectomy

Polypectomy is performed using a wire snare or forceps according to the size of the polyp. It should be kept in mind that bleeding and perforation may occur after polypectomy [23].

4.5 Dilation and stent

Esophageal stricture dilation may be performed using bougie dilators, wire-guided dilators, or balloons. Using the same principles for esophageal stricture dilation, through-the-scope (TTS) balloons can be employed for strictures in the pylorus and duodenum. Stent is an effective method in esophageal malignant strictures and perforations [23].

4.6 Placement of feeding or drainage tubes

Percutaneous endoscopic gastrostomy (PEG) or percutaneous endoscopic jejunostomy (PEJ) can be placed for nutritional purposes. Pancreatic pseudocysts can be drained [2, 23].

4.7 Ablation

Ablation of mucosal lesions of the UGI tract can be performed with a variety of devices including heater probes, multipolar electrocoagulation, argon plasma coagulation (APC), radiofrequency ablation (RFA), neodymium-doped yttrium aluminum garnet (Nd-YAG) laser, cryotherapy [22, 23].

4.8 Achalasia

Pneumatic dilatation, botulinum toxin injection and peroral endoscopic myotomy (POEM) are endoscopic methods used to treat achalasia [24].

4.9 Obesity

Endoscopic sleeve gastroplasti (ESG), intragastric injection of botulinum toxin and gastric balloon is endoscopic weight loss procedures [25].

5. Lower gastrointestinal system endoscopy (colonoscopy) indications

Colonoscopy has largely replaced radiological methods in the diagnosis of lower gastrointestinal system diseases. In addition, taking tissue samples for pathological studies and endoscopic treatment of some diseases are another advantage of colonoscopy. Colonoscopy indications; It is divided into three as diagnostic, follow-up and therapeutic (**Table 2**).

5.1 Diagnostic colonoscopy

5.1.1 Diagnosis of colorectal polyps and cancer

Polyps appear as protrusions of the colon mucosa. Polyps detected during colonoscopy are defined as pedunculated, sessile, flat and depressed. Localization, external structure, size of the detected cancers, whether they prevent the passage of the device or not should be specified [26–28].

Diagnostic	Follow-up	Therapeutic
Colorectal polyps/cancer	Polyps	Foreign body
Rectal bleeding	After colorectal cancer resection	Anastomotic strictures
Chronic diarrhea	Dysplasia	Hemostasis in colorectal bleeding
Iron deficiency anemia	Families with FAP	Endoskopic resections
Changes in bowel habits/ abdominal pain		Volvulus detorsion
Colitis/IBD		Bridging obstructive tumors
Radiological abnormal findings		Polypectomy
Digestive system symptoms		

FAP: Familial adenomatous polyposis, IBD: Inflammatory bowel disease.

Table 2.
Lower gastrointestinal system endoscopy indications.

5.1.2 Rectal bleeding

Melena is generally an indication for gastroscopy, but colonoscopy should be performed if the gastroscopy was nondiagnostic. Hematochezia is usually caused by a lower GI lesion and is often an indication for colonoscopy [29].

5.1.3 Chronic diarrhea

A biopsy by colonoscopy in patients with chronic diarrhea is valuable for the diagnosis of inflammatory diseases and colorectal neoplasia [30].

5.1.4 Iron deficiency anemia

Asymptomatic colonic and gastric carcinoma may present with Iron defiency anemia. Therefore, colonoscopy should be performed together with gastroscopy in patients with iron deficiency anemia [31].

5.1.5 Change In bowel habits, unexplained abdominal pain

Especially in young patients, colonoscopy can be performed to evaluate suspected irritable bowel syndrome if there is abdominal pain and changes in bowel habits [32].

5.1.6 Diagnosis of ulcerative colitis, Crohn's disease, ischemic colitis or other colitis

Colitis can be diagnosed by the characteristic and distribution of lesions or by colonoscopic biopsies. In colitis, ileum cannulation is recommended [33].

5.1.7 Radiologically determined tumor, stenosis, ulcer, diagnosis of lesions such As obstruction

Colonic abnormalities such as colon polyps, mass, focal wall thickening or stenosis identified by X-ray (barium enema) or abdominal computed tomography should be evaluated by colonoscopy [34].

5.1.8 Explaining the findings of patients with digestive system symptoms (such as anorexia, fatigue, weight loss)

Colonoscopy should be performed to explain the findings of especially elderly patients (>50) with digestive system symptoms [35].

5.2 Follow-up colonoscopy

5.2.1 Surveillance of colorectal polyps

Patients with 1–4 < 10 mm adenomas with low-grade dysplasia or serrated polyps <10 mm without dysplasia, regardless of villous components, do not require endoscopic surveillance. Surveillance colonoscopy is recommended after 3 years for patients with at least 1 adenoma ≥10 mm or high-grade dysplasia or ≥ 5 adenomas or any serrated polyp ≥10 mm or dysplasia. If there is a partial endoscopic resection of polyps ≥20 mm, early repeat colonoscopy should be performed at a 3–6 months [36].

5.2.2 Recurrent tumor follow-up after colorectal cancer resection

The first surveillance colonoscopies of patients who have undergone curative resection for colorectal cancer should be scheduled 1 year after surgery. If no neoplastic lesion is detected after the first surveillance colonoscopy following CRC surgery, it would be appropriate to perform the second colonoscopy 3 years later and the third colonoscopy 5 years after the second [37].

5.2.3 Dysplasia follow-up of long-standing ulcerative colitis or Crohn's colitis

Patients with ulcerative colitis or chron colitis whose dysplastic lesions have been completely removed should have endoscopic surveillance at 1 to 6 months and 12 months, and then annual surveillance [38].

5.2.4 Follow-up of families with familial adenomatous polyposis

Colonoscopy surveillance should be planned from the age of 12–14 years in asymptomatic individuals with familial adenomatous polyposis. In patients with familial adenomatous polyposis with an intact colon, colonoscopy surveillance should be performed every 1–2 years, depending on the polyp load [39].

5.3 Therapeutic colonoscopy

5.3.1 Foreign body removal

Foreign body can be removed from the colon utilizing baskets, snares, or biopsy forceps.

5.3.2 Expansion of anastomotic strictures

Balloon dilatation, endoscopic stenosis or stent placement can be performed endoscopically in anastomotic strictures after colorectal surgery [40].

5.3.3 Hemostasis in colorectal bleeding (ulcer, tumor, vascular anomaly, varicose veins, polyps, hemorrhoids)

Lower gastrointestinal bleeding can be treated colonoscopically with electrocoagulation, argon plasma coagulation, injection or band ligation [41].

5.3.4 Endoscopic resections (endoscopic mucosal resection (EMR), endoscopic submucosal dissection (ESD))

Colonic and rectal superficial lesions can be removed curatively by EMR. ESD can be considered for the removal of colon and rectal lesions with a high suspicion of submucosal invasion [42].

5.3.5 Volvulus Detorsion

For patients with uncomplicated sigmoid volvulus the first method of treatment is colonoscopic detorsion and placement of a decompression tube should be considered to prevent repeat volvulus [43].

5.3.6 Bridging obstructive tumors

Colonic stenting may be considered in patients with clinical symptoms and radiological signs of malignant large bowel obstruction and without signs of perforation. Stenting is an alternative way to emergency surgery as a bridge [44].

5.3.7 Polypectomies

Cold snare polypectomy is preferred for the removal of small polyps (size ≤5 mm) and sessile polyps (6–9 mm). When removing sessile polyps larger than 1 cm, submucosal injection can be done due to the risk of thermal injury. It would be appropriate to perform a hot snare polypectomy for pedunculated polyps [45].

The chapter is aimed to review the indications of upper and lower gastrointestinal system endoscopy. The title is "Upper and Lower Gastrointestinal System Endoscopy Indications". Indications for upper gastrointestinal endoscopy (gastroscopy) have increased with the widespread use of flexible endoscopes. Indications for gastroscopy are examined as diagnosis, control, and treatment. In addition, colonoscopy has largely replaced radiological methods in the diagnosis of lower gastrointestinal system diseases. Additionally, taking tissue samples for pathological studies and endoscopic treatment of some diseases are another advantage of colonoscopy. Indications for colonoscopy are examined as diagnosis, control, and treatment. The authors summarize the indications of upper gastrointestinal system endoscopy including diagnostic gastroscopy, control gastroscopy, and the treatment of gastroscopy as well as the indications of lower gastrointestinal system endoscopy (colonoscopy) including diagnostic colonoscopy, control colonoscopy, and the treatment of colonoscopy.

6. Conclusion

In conclusion, endoscopy has a broad range of indications. It is used to confirm or exclude a particular diagnosis in patients with gastrointestinal complaints, to monitor the progression of a known disease, and for staging in patients with a systemic disease.

Author details

Bahadir Kartal[1*] and Mehmet Abdussamet Bozkurt[2]

1 Department of General Surgery, Hitit University Erol Olçok Training and Research Hospital, Corum, Turkey

2 Department of General Surgery, Istinye University, Istanbul, Turkey

*Address all correspondence to: dr.bkartal@hotmail.com

References

[1] ASGE Standards of Practice Committee. The role of endoscopy in dyspepsia. Gastrointestinal Endoscopy. 2007;**66**:1071-1075

[2] Arslan K. Üst Gastrointestinal Sistem Endoskopisi Endikasyonları. In: Karahan Ö, Cingi A, editör. Gastrointestinal Sistem Endoskopisi. 1. Baskı. Ankara: Türk Cerrahi Derneği; 2016.p. 75-79

[3] Wo JM, Mendez C, Harrell S, et al. Clinical impact of upper endoscopy in the management of patients with gastroesophageal reflux disease. The American Journal of Gastroenterology. 2004;**99**:2311-2316

[4] Gralnek IM, Barkun AN, Bardou M. Management of acute bleeding from a peptic ulcer. The New England Journal of Medicine. 2008;**359**:928-937

[5] Navaneethan U, Eubanks S. Approach to patients with esophageal dysphagia. Surgical Clinics of North America. 2015;**95**(3):483-489

[6] Tytgat GNJ. Upper Gastrointestinal Endoscopy, Textbook of Gastroenterology. New York, USA: Lippincott Williams & Wilkins; 1999. pp. 2668-2673

[7] Jacobson BC, Hirota W, Baron TH, et al. ASGE. Obscure gastrointestinal bleeding. Gastrointestinal Endoscopy. 2003;**57**:817-822

[8] Vaezi MF, Pandolfino JE, Vela MF. ACG clinical guideline: Diagnosis and management of achalasia. The American Journal of Gastroenterology. 2013;**108**:1238-1249 quiz 1250

[9] American Society for Gastrointestinal Endoscopy. The role of endoscopy in the surveillance of premalignant conditions of the upper gastrointestinal tract. Gastrointestinal Endoscopy. 1998;**48**:663-668

[10] Sampliner RE. Updated guidelines for the diagnosis, surveillance, and therapy of Barrett's esophagus. The American Journal of Gastroenterology. 2002;**97**:1888-1895

[11] Schnell TG, Sontag SJ, Chejfec G, et al. Long-term nonsurgical management of Barrett's esophagus with high grade dysplasia. Gastroenterology. 2001;**120**:1607-1619

[12] Hirota WK, Zuckerman MJ, Adler DG, et al. Standards of practice committee, American Society for Gastrointestinal Endoscopy. ASGE guideline: The role of endoscopy in the surveillance of premalignant conditions of the upper GI tract. Gastrointestinal Endoscopy. 2006;**63**:570-580

[13] Lundegårdh G, Adami HO, Helmick C, et al. Stomach cancer after partial gastrectomy for benign ulcer disease. The New England Journal of Medicine. 1988;**319**:195-200

[14] ASGE Standards of Practice Committee. Role of endoscopy in the bariatric surgery patient. Gastrointestinal Endoscopy. 2008;**68**:1-10

[15] Kokkola A, Sjoblom S-M, Haapiainen R, et al. The risk of gastric carcinoma and carcinoid tumors in patients with pernicious anemia: A prospective follow-up study. Scandinavian Journal of Gastroenterology. 1998;**33**:88-92

[16] Attard T, Yardley J, Cuffari C. Gastric polyps in pediatrics: An 18 year

hospital based analysis. Am J Gastro. 2002;**97**:298-301

[17] Nakamura S, Matsumoto T, Kobori Y, et al. Impact of helicobacter pylori infection and mucosal atrophy on gastric lesions in patient with familial adenomatous polyposis. Gut. 2002;**51**:485-489

[18] Spigelman AD, Williams CB, Talbot IC, et al. Upper gastrointestinal cancer in patients with familial adenomatous polyposis. Lancet. 1989;**2**:783-785

[19] Watson P, Lynch HT. Extracolonic cancer in hereditary nonpolyposis colorectal cancer. Cancer. 1993;**71**:677-685

[20] Schulman K, Brasch FE, Kunstmann E, et al. HNPCC-associated small bowel cancer: Clinical and molecular characteristics. Gastroenterology. 2005;**128**:590-599

[21] Tincani AJ, Brandalise N, Atemani A, et al. Diagnosis of superficial esophageal cancer and dysplasia using endoscopic screening with a 2% Lugol dye solution in patients with head and neck cancer. Head & Neck. 2000;**22**:170-174

[22] ASGE Standards of Practice Committee. Adverse events of upper GI endoscopy. Gastrointestinal Endoscopy. 2012;**76**:707

[23] Kadayifci A, Brugge WR. Upper gastrointestinal endoscopy. In: Podolsky DK, Camilleri M, Fitz JG, Kalloo AN, Shanahan F, Wang TC, editors. Yamada's Textbook of Gastroenterology. 6 th ed. West Sussex: John Wiley & Sons, Ltd.; 2016. pp. 2552-2557

[24] Khashab MA, Vela MF, Thosani N, et al. ASGE guideline on the management of achalasia. Gastrointestinal Endoscopy. 2020;**91**:213-27.e6

[25] Sampath K, Dinani AM, Rothstein RI. Endoscopic devices for obesity. Current Obesity Reports. 2016;**5**:251-261

[26] Çakır M. Alt Gastrointestinal Sistem Endoskopisi Endikasyonları. In: Karahan Ö, Cingi A, editör. Gastrointestinal Sistem Endoskopisi. 1.Baskı. Ankara: Türk Cerrahi Derneği; 2016.p. 309-310

[27] Lee JM, Cheon JH, Park JJ, et al. Effects of Hyosine N-butyl bromide on the detection of polyps during colonoscopy. Hepato-Gastroenterology. 2010;**57**:90

[28] East JE, Bassett P, Arebi N, et al. Dynamic patient position changes during colonoscope withdrawal increase adenoma detection: A randomized, crossover trial. Gastrointestinal Endoscopy. 2011;**73**:456

[29] Cappell MS, Friedel D. The role of sigmoidoscopy and colonoscopy in the diagnosis and management of lower gastrointestinal disorders: Technique, indications, and contraindications. The Medical Clinics of North America. 2002;**86**:1217-1252

[30] Shen B, Khan K, Ikenberry SO, Anderson MA, Banerjee S, Baron T, et al. The role of endoscopy in the management of patients with diarrhea. Gastrointestinal Endoscopy. 2010;**71**(6):887-892

[31] James MW, Chen CM, Goddard WP, et al. Risk factors for gastrointestinal malignancy in patients with iron-deficiency anaemia. European Journal of Gastroenterology & Hepatology. 2005;**17**:1197e203

[32] Rothstein RD. Irritable bowel syndrome. The Medical Clinics of North America. 2000;**84**:1247-1257

[33] Shergill AK, Lightdale JR, Bruining DH, Acosta RD, Chandrasekhara V, et al. American Society for Gastrointestinal Endoscopy standards of practice committee the role of endoscopy in inflammatory bowel disease. Gastrointestinal Endoscopy. 2015;**81**(5):1101e1-1101e112113

[34] Waye JD, Williams CB. Colonoscopy and flexible sigmoidoscopy. In: Yamada T, Alpers DH, Laine L, et al., editors. Textbook of Gastroenterology. 3rd ed. Philadelphia: Lippincott, Williams & Wilkins; 1999. pp. 2701-2717

[35] Centers for Disease Control and Prevention (CDC). Vital signs: Colorectal cancer screening test use-United States, 2012. MMWR. Morbidity and Mortality Weekly Report. 2013;**62**:881-888

[36] Hassan C, Quintero E, Dumonceau J-M, Regula J, Bretthauer M, Chaussade S, et al. Post-polypectomy colonoscopy surveillance: European Society of Gastrointestinal Endoscopy (ESGE) guideline—Update 2020. Endoscopy. 2020;**52**:687-700

[37] Hassan C, Wysocki PT, Fuccio L, Seufferlein T, Dinis-Ribeiro M, Brandao C, et al. Endoscopic surveillance after surgical or endoscopic resection for colorectal cancer: European Society of Gastrointestinal Endoscopy (ESGE) and European Society of Digestive Oncology (ESDO) guideline. Endoscopy. 2019;**51**:266-277. DOI: 10.1055/a-0831-2522

[38] American Society for Gastrointestinal Endoscopy Standards of Practice Committee, Shergill AK, Lightdale JR, Bruining DH, Acosta RD, Chandrasekhara V, et al. The role of endoscopy in inflammatory bowel disease. Gastrointestinal Endoscopy. 2015;**81**:1101-21.e1

[39] Van Leerdam ME, Roos VH, Van Hooft JE, et al. Endoscopic management of polyposis syndromes: European Society of Gastrointestinal Endoscopy (ESGE) guideline. Endoscopy. 2019;**51**:877-895

[40] Zhang LJ, Lan N, Wu XR, Shen B. Endoscopic stricturotomy in the treatment of anastomotic strictures in inflammatory bowel disease (IBD) and non-IBD patients. Gastroenterol Rep (Oxf). 2020;**8**:143-150

[41] Rubin PH, Naymagon S, Williams CB, Waye JD. Colonoscopy and flexible sigmoidoscopy. In: Podolsky DK, Camilleri M, Fitz JG, Kalloo AN, Shanahan F, Wang TC, editors. Yamada's Textbook of Gastroenterology. 6th ed. West Sussex: John Wiley & Sons, Ltd.; 2016. pp. 2569-2581

[42] Pimentel-Nunes P et al. Endoscopic submucosal dissection: European Society of Gastrointestinal Endoscopy (ESGE) guideline. Endoscopy. 2015;**47**:829-854. DOI: 10.1055/s-0034-1392882

[43] Naveed M, Jamil LH, Fuji-Lau LL, et al. American Society for Gastrointestinal Endoscopy guideline on the role of endoscopy in the management of acute colonic pseudo-obstruction and colonic volvulus. Gastrointestinal Endoscopy. 2020;**91**:228-235. DOI: 10.1016/j.gie.2019.09.007

[44] van Hooft JE, Veld JV, Arnold D, et al. Self-expandable metal stents for obstructing colonic and extracolonic cancer: European Society of Gastrointestinal Endoscopy (ESGE) guideline – Update 2020. Endoscopy. 2020;**52**:389-407

[45] Ferlitsch M, Moss A, Hassan C, et al. Colorectal polypectomy and endoscopic mucosal resection (EMR): European Society of Gastrointestinal Endoscopy (ESGE) clinical guideline. Endoscopy. 2017;**49**:270-297

Chapter 2

Efficacy of Holmium Laser Enucleation of the Prostate in Men with Bladder Outlet Obstruction and Intravesical Prostatic Protrusion: A Functional View

Lorenzo Capone

Abstract

The principal aim of this chapter is to evaluate the urodynamic and clinical outcomes at 6 months follow-up in men with or without significant IPP (> 5 mm) undergoing HoLEP for BOO. Eight-four patients underwent HoLEP between January 2018 and December 2021. Inclusion criteria: men aged 50–75 years with prostate size from 30 to 100 grams, peak urinary flow rate less than 15 ml/s, and a diagnosis of BOO. At 6-month follow-up, urodynamics data show a statistically significant reduction in PdetOpen and PdetQmax compared with baseline in both IPP and no IPP groups. Statistically significant differences were found in maximal urodynamic bladder capacity before and after the operations in both groups as also IPSS data, Qmax, Qave, PVR and IPSS total score at 6 months when compared with preoperative data. HoLEP is efficient in improving functional outcomes and obstructive symptoms regardless of the presence of IPP. Surgeons can expect better postoperative outcomes in terms of Qmax, Qave and IPSS total score in patients with significant IPP.

Keywords: bladder outlet obstruction, benign prostatic hyperplasia surgical treatment, urodynamic study, functional urology

1. Introduction

Lower urinary tract symptoms (LUTS) have traditionally been related to bladder outlet obstruction (BOO), which is often caused by benign prostatic enlargement (BPE) resulting from the histologic condition of benign prostatic hyperplasia (BPH) [1, 2]. Despite bladder dysfunction may cause LUTS as well as other structural or functional abnormalities of the urinary tract, BPH is the major etiology of LUTS in men older than 50 years: almost more than 70% of patients greater than 70 years old is affected [2, 3].

Recent studies have emphasized the relationship between prostate configuration and BOO associated with LUTS suggesting the idea of a prostate adenoma arising from nodular hyperplasia that distorts the prostatic urethra rather than compressing it [4–6].

Unlike prostate volume (PV), the intravesical prostatic protrusion (IPP) has been shown that it well correlates with poor urinary flow and the presence of BOO [6, 7]. IPP is a phenomenon in which the prostate adenoma enlarges into the bladder along the plane of least resistance leading to a "ball-valve" type of obstruction, which disrupts the funneling effect of the bladder neck and leads to an uncoordinated movement of the detrusor muscle during voiding [7–9].

Surgical intervention is the standard treatment for patients with bothersome LUTS due to BOO who are unwilling to try medical therapies, both in cases where medical therapies were not effective and in cases of complicated LUTS [10, 11]. Historically, transurethral resection of the prostate (TURP) has been the gold standard to which all endoscopic procedures for BPH are compared, but, in the past 2 decades, a wide range of innovative transurethral procedures have challenged his supremacy. Holmium laser enucleation of the prostate (HoLEP) proposed by Gilling et al. in 1995 [12] seems to be a valid alternative to standard TURP with comparable functional outcomes, symptoms improvement, a shorter catheterization and hospitalization times [13–15].
Urodynamic studies and in particular pression/flow studies can provide objective and crucial diagnostic information before and after the treatment, and there is a general agreement that these studies are the basis to quantify BOOs [16, 17].

The principal aim of this study is to evaluate the urodynamic and clinical outcomes at 6 months follow-up in men with or without significant IPP (>5 mm) undergoing HoLEP for BOO.

2. Material and methods

We enrolled 84 patients who underwent HoLEP at our Institution between January 2018 and January 2021. Inclusion criteria were men aged 50–75 years with prostate size from 30 to 100 g, peak urinary flow rate (Qmax) less than 15 ml/s and a diagnosis of BOO, according to clinical symptoms, and related examinations. Exclusion criteria were patients with urologic tumors, uncontrolled diabetes, neurogenic bladder, previous radiation therapy and patients who refused to agree with the informed consent.

All patients underwent a preoperative examination with anamnesis, digital rectal examination, urinalysis, uroflowmetry (URF), trans abdominal ultrasonography with IPP evaluation, postvoid residual urine volume (PVR), blood analysis with prostate specific antigen (PSA) and a urodynamic study with pression/flow study (UDS). All patients compiled the International Prostate Symptoms Score (IPSS).

Operation indications were medical therapy failure, refusal of medical treatment and a BOO diagnosed by UDS. All patients performed an outpatient visit, URF, UDS, PVR and IPSS after 6 months from the operation.

3. IPP measurements and grading

For the assessment of the IPP most of the studies use transabdominal ultrasound with a bladder capacity between 150 and 250 ml. IPP was defined as the vertical distance from the tip of the intravesical protrusion to the bladder circumference at the base of the prostate gland. With respect to these measurements, the grading system was: Grade I < 5 mm; Grade II 5–10 mm; Grade III > 10 mm. The literature agrees that Grade II and III are correlated to severe BOO, and this has been considered as positive in our study [7, 18].

We divided the patients into two groups based on the IPP: patients with bladders with IPP of 5 or less were assigned to group 1 (no IPP group) and patients with IPP of 6 or more were assigned to group 2 (IPP group).

In order to minimize the bias and for more precise IPP measurement the same urologist performed the transabdominal ultrasound with the same device.

4. Urodynamic study

UDS was performed following the recommendation of the International Continence Society, Good Urodynamics Practices and Terms [19] by the same examiner throughout the study period with the same device (SmartDyn, Albyn Medical S.L, Cordovilla, E). The intravesical pressure was measured using a double lumen 6 Ch catheter; the abdominal pressure using a rectal balloon catheter. Cystomanometry was performed with sterile saline solution (0.9%) at 25°C with infusion rate of 50 ml/min. Transducers were balanced at atmospheric zero. The patient was asked to report any sensation relating to bladder filling (first sensation, normal sensation and strong desire to void); the volume at which additional filling was stopped was considered the maximal urodynamic bladder capacity (UBC). During pression/flow study, it was measured the detrusor pressure at urethral opening pressure (Pdet Open) at maximum flow (Pdet Qmax), and it was plotted on two graphics: the Schafer and the ICS nomograms, in order to evaluate the degree of obstruction and the detrusor strength. The UDS was performed before the operation and after a 6-months follow-up.

5. HoLEP technique

The surgical technique used for the enucleation of the prostate was the same first described by Gilling et al [12]. The holmium laser energy was delivered by a 550-micron fiber placed in a 24 Ch resectoscope and the same urologist performed enucleation with a high-power holmium laser (100-Watt platform, Lumenis). The settings were 2.0 J energy and 40–50 Hz frequency; hemostasis settings were 1.5 J and 30 Hz with a wide pulse. Once enucleation was completed, the inner laser sheath was replaced with a straight nephroscope and a morcellator was introduced. This was used to extract the prostate tissue once the bladder had been fully distended using dual inflows. After the procedure, a 22 Ch 3-way silicon Dufour was used and catheterization time, hospital stay, and hemoglobin were recorded.

6. Statistical analysis

Statistical analysis was performed using the Statistical Package for the Social Sciences (SPSS), version 26.0 (SPSS Inc., Chicago, IL). p-Values <0.05 were considered statistically significant. Student t-test was used for the comparison between means of independent groups, and 2-tailed t-test for paired samples. All patients provided written informed consent.

7. Results

Among 84 patients who underwent HoLEP, 41 were included in group 1 (IPP $\leq$ 5 mm) and 43 in group 2 (IPP > 5 mm). The mean patients age was 63.3 $\pm$ 5.3.

In line with Schafer and ICS nomograms all patients were obstructed at baseline (Schafer > 2, "Obstructed" in accordance with ICS). There were statistically significant differences between IPP and no IPP groups in terms of mean serum PSA level and PV (IPP: 2.9 ± 0.5 ng/mL, 68.2 ± 9.0 g; no IPP: 2.0 ± 0.3 ng/mL, 53.9 ± 5.3 g; $p < 0.001$). There was also a significant difference between the two groups in terms of IPSS total score during the outpatient visit before the operations (IPP: 26.1 ± 1.5; no IPP 23.1 ± 0.8; $p < 0.001$).

As far as it concerns the operative and post-operative data, the overall operative time was significantly longer in the IPP group (IPP: 81.3 ± 12.4 min; no IPP 72.4 ± 5.4; $p < 0.05$) and the catheterization time that was slightly lower in no IPP group (IPP: 107.2 h ± 12.2 h; no IPP: 96 ± 7.4 h; $p < 0.003$). Blood loss and general hospital stay were equivalent in both groups and not statistically significant as the surgical complications (**Table 1**). After the operation, all patients were dismissed with antibiotic therapy to minimize the irritative symptoms related to the procedure.

At 6 months follow up, urodynamics data show a statistically significant reduction in PdetOpen and PdetQmax compared with baseline in both IPP and no IPP groups (IPP: PdetOpen preop 89.8 ± 16 cmH_2O, 6-mo 34.5 ± 6.9 cmH_2O; no IPP: PdetOpen preop 64.5 ± 11.8 cmH_2O, 6-mo 34.8 ± 5.9 cmH_2O. IPP: PdetQmax preop 102.5 ± 17.6 cmH_2O, 6-mo 36.6 ± 7.1 cmH_2O; no IPP: PdetQmax preop 77.5 ± 12.6 cmH_2O, 6-mo 38.8 ± 5.2 cmH_2O; $p < 0.001$). Also, the Schafer and ICS nomograms confirm the effectiveness of HoLEP in improving functional outcomes in both all IPP and no IPP patients (Schafer < 2, "Non obstructed" in accordance with ICS). Statistically significant differences were found in maximal UBC before and after the operations in both groups (IPP postop + 38.1 ± 19.2: no IPP post + 18.7 ± 9.4) as also IPSS data, Qmax, Qave, PVR and IPSS total score at 6-months when compared with preoperative data (**Table 2**, $p < 0.001$).

A comparison was also made between IPP and no IPP group patients before and after surgery with statistically significant differences. IPP group had a higher IPSS total score, PdetOpen and PdetQmax at baseline (IPP vs. no IPP: PdetOpen 89.8 ± 16.0 vs. 64.5 ± 11.8 cmH_2O; PdetQmax 102.5 ± 17.6 vs. 77.5 ± 12.6 cmH_2O,

Characteristic	IPP	No IPP	*p*-Value
No. of patients	43	41	/
Age (year)	63.87 ± 5.89	67.77 ± 4.78	/
Total PSA (ng/ml)	2.89 ± 0.55	2.01 ± 0.26	<0.001
Prostate volume (g)	68.20 ± 9.08	53.92 ± 5.31	<0.001
IPSS total score	26.06 ± 1.58	21.23 ± 5.89	<0.001
Total operative time (min)	81.33 ± 12.46	72.38 ± 5.47	0.24
Hemoglobin (g/dl)			
Preoperative	14.94 ± 0.69	14.23 ± 0.72	0.14
Postoperative	13.96 ± 0.70	13.39 ± 0.68	0.20
Hospital stay (hour)	76.80 ± 9.93	73.22 ± 5.08	0.09
Catheterization time (hour)	107.28 h ± 12.38	96.48 ± 7.41	<0.003

Table 1.
Patient characteristics and perioperative outcomes.

$p < 0.001$; IPSS score 26.1 ± 1.6 vs. 21.2 ± 5.9, $p < 0.05$) associated with a lower maximal UBC (IPP vs. no IPP: 316.6 ± 35.1 vs. 371.3 ± 45.6 ml; $p < 0.01$). Furthermore, the IPP group was associated with a higher postoperative Qave, Qmax

Pdet Qmax (cmH_2O)			
	IPP	**No IPP**	***p*-Value**
Baseline	102.53 ± 17.61	77.46 ± 12.62	<0.001
6-Month	36.60 ± 7.16	38.85 ± 5.25	0.39
p-Value	<0.001	<0.001	
Pdet open (cmH_2O)			
	IPP	No IPP	*p*-Value
Baseline	89.8 ± 16.03	64.46 ± 11.81	<0.001
6-Month	34.53 ± 6.93	34.77 ± 5.89	0.92
p-Value	<0.001	<0.001	
UBC (ml)			
	IPP	No IPP	*p*-Value
Baseline	89.8 ± 16.03	64.46 ± 11.81	<0.001
6-Month	34.53 ± 6.93	34.77 ± 5.89	0.045
p-Value	<0.001	<0.001	
Schafer (points)			
	IPP	No IPP	*p*-Value
Baseline	4.67 ± 0.81	4.46 ± 0.52	0.24
6-Month	1.30 ± 0.73	1.55 ± 0.37	0.53
p-Value	<0.001	<0.001	
Qmax (ml/s)			
	IPP	No IPP	*p*-Value
Baseline	7.66 ± 1.99	8.67 ± 2.46	<0.001
6-Month	23.88 ± 2.36	21.11 ± 1.01	<0.001
p-Value	<0.001	<0.001	
Qave (ml/s)			
	IPP	No IPP	*p*-Value
Baseline	2.98 ± 0.92	4.01 ± 1.21	<0.001
6-Month	12.63 ± 1.62	10.24 ± 1.05	<0.001
p-Value	<0.001	<0.001	
PVR (ml)			
	IPP	No IPP	*p*-Value
Baseline	75.33 ± 22.24	70.77 ± 11.15	<0.51
6-Month	38.73 ± 15.94	46.38 ± 8.61	<0.13
p-Value	<0.001	<0.001	

IPSS (points)			
	IPP	No IPP	p-Value
Baseline	26.07 ± 1.58	21.23 ± 5.89	< 0.001
6-Month	3.67 ± 0.81	5.92 ± 0.95	< 0.001
p-Value	<0.001	<0.001	

Table 2.
Urodynamic test outcomes at baseline pre-Holep and 6 months after surgery in patient with significant or nonsignificant IPP.

(IPP vs. no IPP: Qave 12.6 ± 1.6 vs. 10.6 ± 1.1 ml/s; Qmax 23.9 ± 2.4 vs. 21.1 ± 1.0 ml/s; $p < 0.001$) and a lower IPSS total score than the no IPP group (IPP vs. no IPP: IPSS score 3.7 ± 0.8 vs. 5.9 ± 0.9, $p < 0.001$). No statistically significant decrease was observed after 6 months in PdetOpen, PdetQmax and UBC values in IPP group compared to no IPP group (**Table 3**).

8. Discussion

To the best of our knowledge, this is the first study showing the functional outcomes after HoLEP in men with significant IPP and one of the few reports considering postoperative urodynamic data in patients with severe BOO.

We know that BOO results from functional or anatomic etiologies and produces compression or resistance upon the bladder outflow channel at any location from the bladder neck to the urethral meatus. This produces LUTS, which may be predominantly obstructive, irritative, or often a combination of both [20].

As a result of chronic obstruction, the bladder wall is markedly remodeled, including cellular hyspertrophy, hyperplasia, and reorganization of the structural relationship between connective tissue and smooth muscle elements [21, 22]. All these changes lead to an initial detrusor overactivity (DO), but the longer BOO persists, the more function instability remains, ending with a hypo/acontractile bladder [23].

Urodynamics with pressure flow studies remains the gold standard for diagnosing and quantifying BOO [24] because they provide patients with correct information about their recovery in case of DO or reduce the non-necessary number of medical or surgical interventions in case of hypocontractility. For this reason, a urodynamic study is essential for a correct functional assessment in patients with BOO, irrespective of the procedure [19, 25]. Within this context there are several studies that focused not only on the size of the prostate but also on its shape and in particular on the association between IPP and BOO.

Chia et al. in 2003 were the first who demonstrated a correlation between IPP and BOO. They suggested the IPP obstruction as a "ball-valve" type capable of disrupting the funnel effect of bladder neck and causing a dyskinetic movement of the bladder during voiding. IPP in enrolled patients was graded using transabdominal US in 3 groups: grade I (<5 mm), grade II (5–10 mm), grade III (>10 mm). In patients with BOO confirmed on the pressure-flow study, grade III IPP was associated with a higher BOO index (BOOI) than grade I–II ($P < 0.001$) [7]. Keqin et al. in 2007 reported an association between reduced Qmax at URF and severe BOO in significant IPP patients (IPP > 10 mm). They also demonstrated the benefit from early surgical intervention

DOI: http://dx.doi.org/10.5772/intechopen.108388

Pdet Qmax (cmH2O)			
	IPP	No IPP	p Value
Baseline	102	77	< 0.001
6-Month	36	38	0.39
p Value	< 0.001	< 0.001	

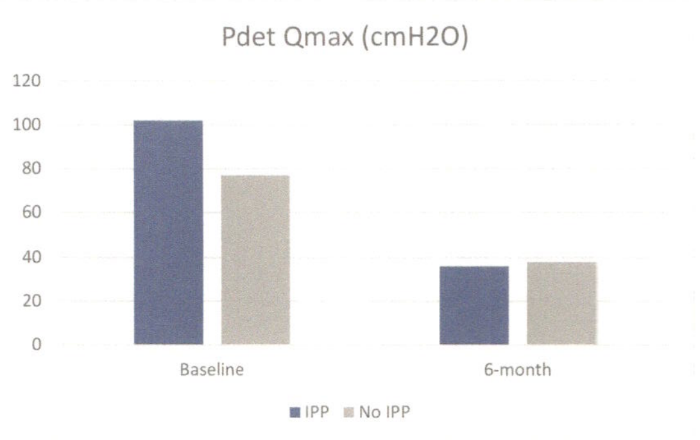

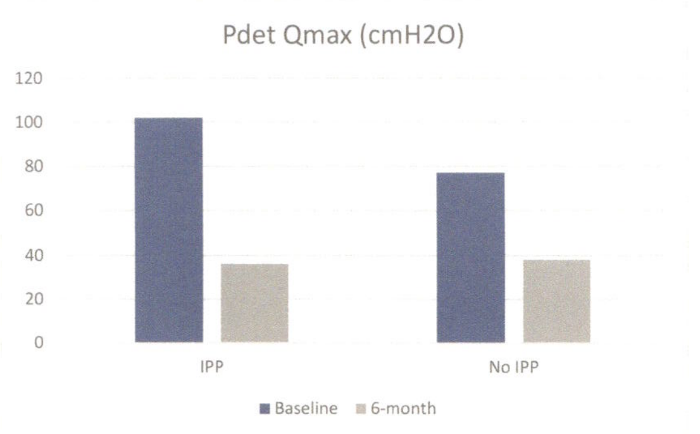

Pdet Open (cmH2O)			
	IPP	No IPP	p Value
Baseline	89	64	< 0.001
6-Month	34	34	0.92
p Value	< 0.001	< 0.001	

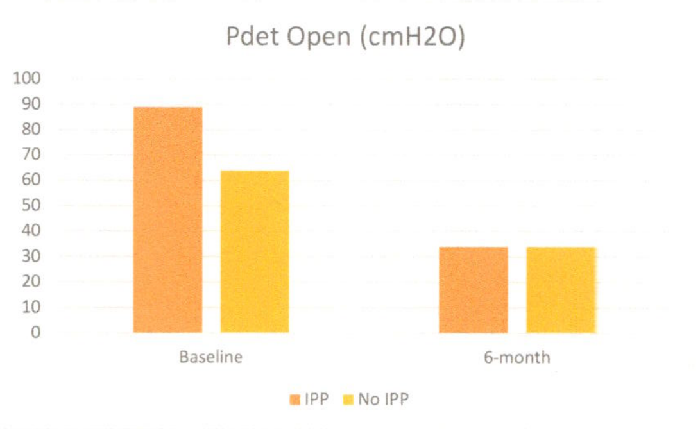

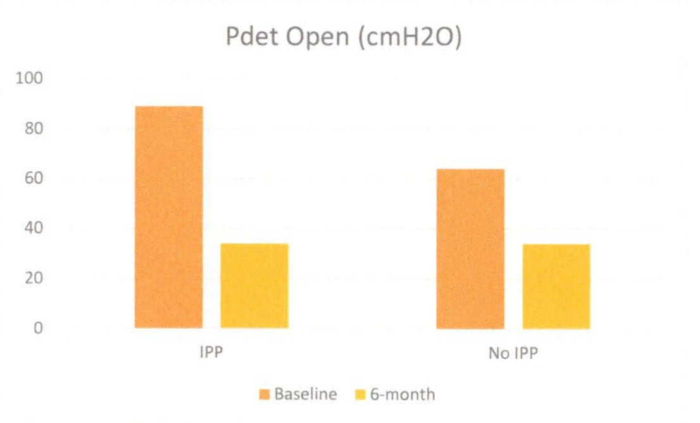

Qmax (ml/s)			
	IPP	No IPP	p Value
Baseline	7	8	< 0.001
6-Month	24	21	< 0.001

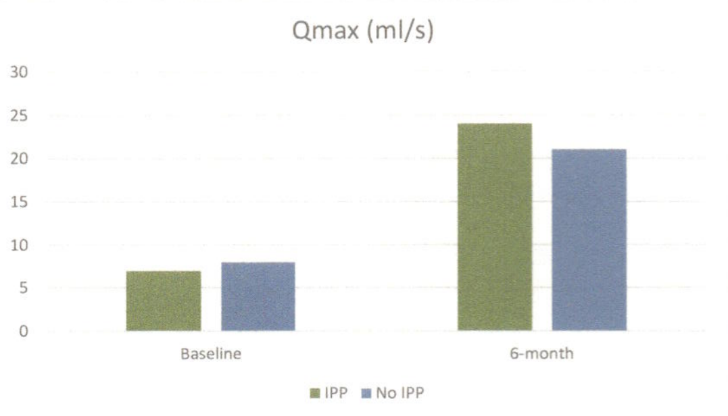

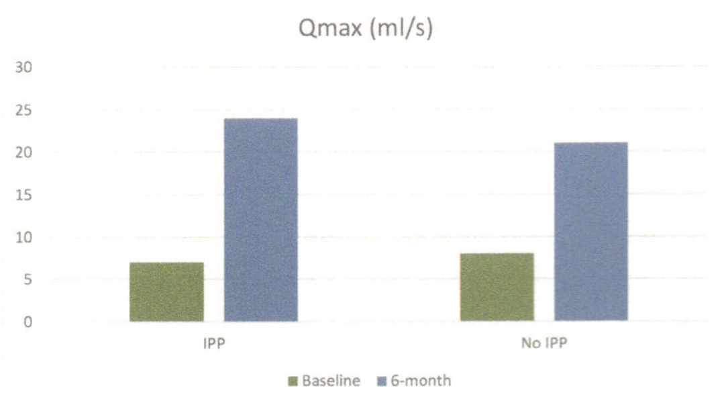

Qave (ml/s)			
	IPP	No IPP	p Value
Baseline	3	4	< 0.001
6-month	12	10	< 0.001
p Value	< 0.001	< 0.001	

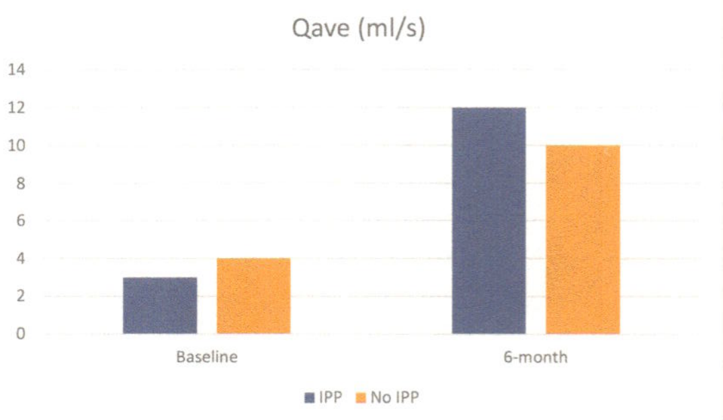

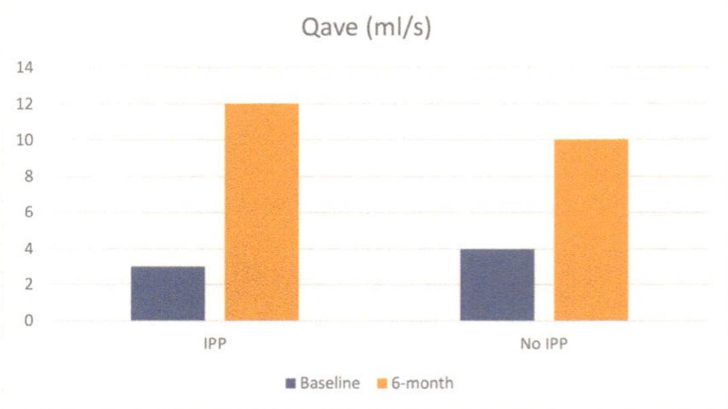

Table 3.
Outcomes between IPP and non-IPP group in terms of PdetQmax, PdetOpen, Qmax and Qave.

in these patients [26]. Rieken et al. in their 2017 systemic review summarized that IPP measured with transabdominal US is a simple and accurate method to predict BOO emphasizing the correlation between an IPP > 10 mm and a reduced Qmax, an increased BOOI and detrusor wall thickness [27].

Other important findings are the strong correlation between high IPP and trial without catheter (TWOC) or medical treatment effect. Mariappan et al. in 2007 [28] studied 121 patients with acute urinary retention related to BPH and receiving alpha-blockers before a TWOC; IPP appears to strongly predict the outcome of a TWOC that was more likely to fail in patients with IPP larger than 10 mm. Another study showed that patients with high grade IPP after an acute urinary retention episode had an unsuccessful TWOC close to 90% [29]. Lee et al. [30] found that patients with IPP grade II–III had a significantly higher risk of clinical progression of BPE after a 32-month follow-up compared to patients with IPP grade I.

Despite the large number of studies correlating high grade IPP with BOO clinical progression, only three studies investigated the presence and degree of IPP with postoperative outcome after BOO surgery.

Lee et al. in 2012 reviewed 177 patients who underwent TURP and followed them after 6-month follow-up. They divided patients into 2 groups—no IPP (<5 mm), IPP (≥5 mm)—and considered IPSS total and partial score (IPSS-voiding; IPSS-storage), QoL, Qmax, PVR and transitional zone volume (TZV). At 6-month follow-up after the surgical procedure IPSS, IPSS-v, IPSS-s and QoL score were better in IPP group, and this concluded that IPP is an independent parameter for predicting postoperative outcomes in BPH patients undergoing TURP [31].

On the other hand, two other studies on patients undergoing photoselective vaporization of the prostate (PVP) with 120 W HPS laser did not find statistically significant differences in outcomes between patients with or without IPP [32]. Kim et al. evaluated the presence of IPP in 134 patients between January 2010 and July 2011 by retroflexed view from flexible cystoscopy (significant IPP > 5 mm). The Qmax was improved in the IPP group (+7.8 ml/L/s) compared with no IPP group (+6.0 ml/s) and in total IPSS, IPSS-v and IPSS-s as well, after 1 and 3 months. The superiority of the IPP group was not sustained at 6-month follow-up [33].

Our study takes into consideration patients subjected to HoLEP that both the EAU and AUA guidelines on the surgical treatment of BPH recommend as a size-independent treatment option for those men with moderate to severe symptoms [11, 34]. In line with the literature, we noticed that patients in the IPP group had a higher serum PSA (+0.88 ng/mL) and IPSS total score (+4.8 points) because of their larger prostatic volume (+14.3 gr). Our study also showed a higher PdetOpen (+25.3 cmH_2O) and PdetQmax (+25.1 cmH_2O) at baseline in IPP patients associated with a lower UBC (−54.7 ml). This data can be explained by the fact that opening bladder neck and urethral channel during micturition is more difficult and requires a more forceful detrusor contraction when there is a middle lobe protrusion causing constriction [35, 36]. We also noticed a dramatic improvement in urodynamics and clinical findings in both groups of patients before the procedure and at 6-month follow up. In particular, pression/flow studies showed that an early diagnosis of BOO due to prostatic obstruction is associated with excellent surgical outcomes regardless the presence of IPP and with a normal detrusor motor activity; most likely because the detrusor did not still have irreversible damage (IPP group Qmax + 16.2 mL/s; PdetQmax – 65.9 cmH_2O; PVR – 35.6 mL; UBC + 38.1 ml. No IPP group Qmax + 12.4 mL/s; PdetQmax – 38.6 cmH_2O; PVR – 24.4 ml; UBC + 18.7 ml. $p < 0.001$) (**Figures 1** and **2**).

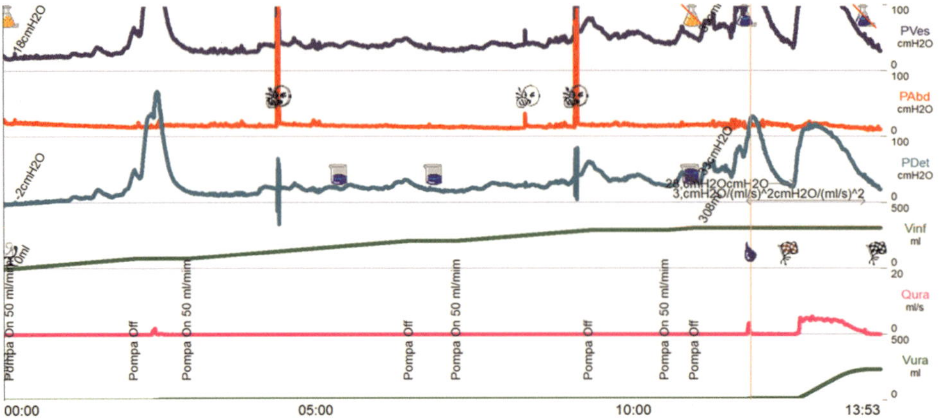

Figure 1.
Urodynamics showing BOO pre-Holep.

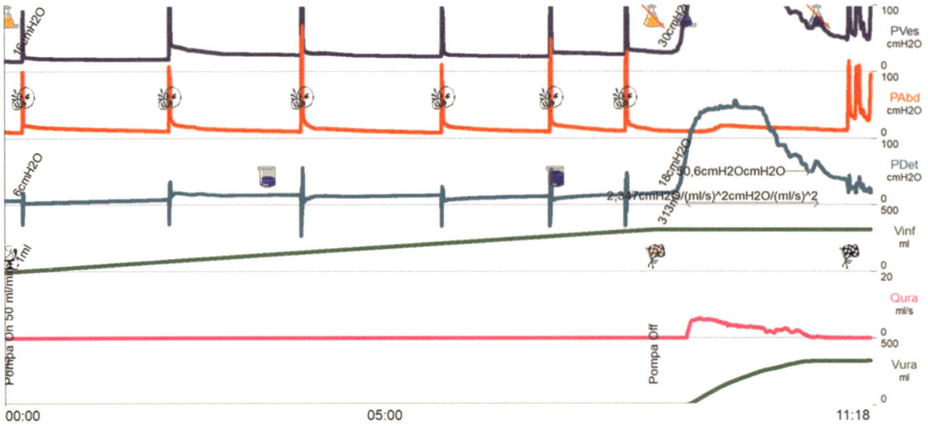

Figure 2.
Normal urodynamics post-Holep.

As regards the functional and clinical outcomes between the two groups at 6-month follow-up, we noticed an increased Qmax (+2.77 ml/s) and Qave (+2.39 ml/s) in the IPP group, but these data were not endorsed by the UDS counterpart that showed non-statistically differences between the two groups. Similar data were published in 2006 by Rigatti et al. [37] who compared urodynamic studies in patients undergoing TURP and HoLEP before and after 1-year follow-up and found PdetQmax value not particularly efficient in describing an effect of surgery on BOO. Lastly, patients with significant IPP experienced less symptoms at 6-month follow-up IPSS total score (−2.26 points) in agreement with Lee and his group [31].

A limitation of this study is the lack of information at a greater distance (1 year), also considering the long-term complications of the procedure like incontinence, urethral stricture, or erectile dysfunction.

9. Conclusions

Our results demonstrated that HoLEP is efficient in improving functional outcomes and obstructive symptoms regardless the presence of IPP. We also show that surgeons can expect better postoperative outcomes in terms of Qmax, Qave and IPSS total score in patients with significant IPP; this likely because a higher detrusor activity without bladder wall irreversible damage had been urodinamically detected.

Author details

Lorenzo Capone
Department of Urology, Fondazione IRCCS Casa Sollievo Della Sofferenza, San Giovanni Rotondo, Italy

*Address all correspondence to: lorenzocapone@msn.com

References

[1] Abrams P et al. The standardisation of terminology of lower urinary tract function: Report from the Standardisation Sub-committee of the International Continence Society. Neurourology and Urodynamics. 2002;**21**:167

[2] Chapple CR et al. Lower urinary tract symptoms revisited: A broader clinical perspective. European Urology. 2008;**54**: 563

[3] Wei JT, Calhoun E, Jacobsen SJ. Urologic diseases in America project: Benign prostatic hyperplasia. Journal of Urology. 2005;**173**(4):1256-1261

[4] Foo KT. Solving the benign prostatic hyperplasia puzzle. Asian Journal of Urology. 2016;**3**:6-9

[5] Sigdel GB, Belokar WK. Clinical significance of intravesical prostatic protrusion in patients with benign prostatic hyperplasia. Journal of Universal College of Medical Sciences. 2015;**3**:6-10

[6] Gandhi J, Weissbart SJ, Kim AN, Joshi G, Kaplan SA, Khan SA. Clinical considerations for intravesical prostatic protrusion in the evaluation and management of bladder outlet obstruction secondary to benign prostatic hyperplasia. Current Urology. 2018 Oct;**12**(1):6-12. DOI: 10.1159/000447224. Epub 2018 Jun 30

[7] Chia SJ, Heng CT, Chan SP, Foo KT. Correlation of intravesical prostatic protrusion with bladder outlet obstruction. BJU International. 2003;**91**: 371-374

[8] Zheng J, Pan J, Qin Y, Huang J, Luo Y, Gao X, et al. Role for intravesical prostatic protrusion in lower urinary tract symptom: A fluid structural interaction analysis study. BMC Urology. 2015;**15**:86

[9] Moss MC, Rezan T, Karaman UR, Gomelsky A. Treatment of concomitant OAB and BPH. Current Urology Reports. 2017;**18**(1):1. DOI: 10.1007/s11934-017-0649-z

[10] McVary KT, Roehrborn CG, Avins AL, Barry MJ, Bruskewitz RC, Donnell RF, et al. Update on AUA guideline on the management of benign prostatic hyperplasia. Journal of Urology. 2011;**185**(5):1793-1803. DOI: 10.1016/j.juro.2011.01.074. Epub 2011 Mar 21

[11] EAU Guidelines: Management of Non-Neurogenic Male Lower Urinary Tract Symptoms (LUTS), incl. Benign Prostatic Obstruction (BPO) Edn. presented at the EAU Annual Congress Amsterdam 2022. ISBN 978-94-92671-16-5

[12] Gilling PJ et al. Combination holmium and Nd:YAG laser ablation of the prostate: Initial clinical experience. Journal of Endourology. 1995;**9**:151

[13] Gilling PJ et al. Long-term results of a randomized trialvcomparing holmium laser enucleation of the prostate and transurethral resection of the prostate: Results at 7 years. BJU International. 2012;**109**(3):408-411

[14] Cornu JN, Ahyai S, Bachmann A, de la Rosette J, Gilling P, Gratzke C, et al. A systematic review and meta-analysis of functional outcomes and complications following transurethral procedures for lower urinary tract symptoms resulting from benign prostatic obstruction: An update. European Urology. 2015;**67**(6): 1066-1096. DOI: 10.1016/j.eururo.2014.06.017. Epub 2014 Jun 25

[15] Das AK, Teplitsky S, Humphreys MR. Holmium laser enucleation of the prostate (HoLEP): A review and update. Canadian Journal of Urology. 2019;**26**(4 Suppl 1):13-19

[16] Griffiths DJ. Pressure-flow studies of micturition. Urologic Clinics of North America. 1996;**23**(2):279-297. DOI: 10.1016/s0094-0143(05)70311-6

[17] Clement KD et al. Invasive urodynamic studies for the management of lower urinary tract symptoms (LUTS) in men with voiding dysfunction. Cochrane Database of Systematic Reviews. 2015:CD011179

[18] Franco G, De Nunzio C, Leonardo C, Tubaro A, Ciccariello M, De Dominicis C, et al. Ultrasound assessment of intravesical prostatic protrusion and detrusor wall thickness—New standards for noninvasive bladder outlet obstruction diagnosis? Journal of Urology. 2010;**183**(6):2270-2274. DOI: 10.1016/j.juro.2010.02.019. Epub 2010 Apr 18

[19] Rosier PFWM, Schaefer W, Lose G, Goldman HB, Guralnick M, Eustice S, et al. International Continence Society Good Urodynamic Practices and Terms 2016: Urodynamics, uroflowmetry, cystometry, and pressure-flow study. Neurourology and Urodynamics. 2017; **36**(5):1243-1260. DOI: 10.1002/nau.23124. Epub 2016 Dec 5

[20] Dmochowsk RR. Bladder outlet obstruction: Etiology and evaluation. Revista de Urología. 2005;7(Suppl. 6): S3-S13

[21] Levin RM, Haugaard N, O'Connor L, Buttyan R, Das A, Dixon JS, et al. Obstructive response of human bladder to BPH vs. rabbit bladder response to partial outlet obstruction: A direct comparison. Neurourology and Urodynamics. 2000;**19**:609-629

[22] Mirone V, Imbimbo C, Longo N, Fusco F. The detrusor muscle: An innocent victim of bladder outlet obstruction. European Urology. 2007;**51**: 57-66

[23] Agartan CA, Whitbeck C, Chichester P, Kogan BA, Levin RM. Effect of age on rabbit bladder function and structure following partial outlet obstruction. Journal of Urology. 2005; **173**:1400-1405

[24] Nitti VW. Pressure flow urodynamic studies: The gold standard for diagnosing bladder outlet obstruction. Revista de Urología. 2005;7(Suppl. 6):S14-S21

[25] Abrams P, Cardozo L, Fall M, Griffiths D, Rosier P, Ulmsten U, et al. Standardisation Sub-Committee of the International Continence Society. The standardisation of terminology in lower urinary tract function: Report from the standardisation sub-committee of the International Continence Society. Urology. 2003;**61**(1):37-49. DOI: 10.1016/s0090-4295(02)02243-4

[26] Keqin Z, Zhishun X, Jing Z, Haixin W, Dongqing Z, Benkang S. Clinical significance of intravesical prostatic protrusion in patients with benign prostatic enlargement. Urology. 2007;**70**:1096-1099

[27] Rieken M, Presicce F, Autorino R, Nunzio DE, C. Clinical significance of intravesical prostatic protrusion in the management of benign prostatic enlargement: A systematic review and critical analysis of current evidence. Minerva Urologica e Nefrologica. 2017; **69**(6):548-555. DOI: 10.23736/S0393-2249.17.02828-4

[28] Mariappan P, Brown DJ, McNeill AS. Intravesical prostatic protrusion is better than prostate volume in predicting the outcome of trial without catheter in

white men presenting with acute urinary retention: A prospective clinical study. Journal of Urology. 2007;**178**(2):573-577; discussion 577. DOI: 10.1016/j.juro.2007.03.116. Epub 2007 Jun 14

[29] Mehraban D. Clinical value of intravesical prostatic protrusion in the evaluation and management of prostatic and other lower urinary tract diseases. Asian Journal of Urology. 2017;**4**(3):174-180. DOI: 10.1016/j.ajur.2016.10.001. Epub 2017 Jan 20

[30] Lee LS, Sim HG, Lim KB, Wang D, Foo KT. Intravesical prostatic protrusion predicts clinical progression of benign prostatic enlargement in patients receiving medical treatment. International Journal of Urology. 2010;**17**(1):69-74. DOI: 10.1111/j.1442-2042.2009.02409.x. Epub 2009 Nov 16

[31] Lee JW, Ryu JH, Yoo TK, Byun SS, Jeong YJ, Jung TY. Relationship between intravesical prostatic protrusion and postoperative outcomes in patients with benign prostatic hyperplasia. Korean Journal of Urology. 2012;**53**(7):478-482. DOI: 10.4111/kju.2012.53.7.478. Epub 2012 Jul 19

[32] Kang SH, Choi YS, Kim SJ, Cho HJ, Hong SH, Lee JY, et al. Long-term follow-up results of photoselective vaporization of the prostate with the 120 W greenlight HPS laser for treatment of benign prostatic hyperplasia. Korean Journal of Urology. 2011;**52**(4):260-264. DOI: 10.4111/kju.2011.52.4.260. Epub 2011 Apr 22

[33] Kim MS, Park KK, Chung BH, Lee SH. Effect of photoselective vaporization prostatectomy on lower urinary tract symptoms in benign prostatic hyperplasia with or without intravesical prostatic protrusion. Korean Journal of Urology. 2013;**54**(1):36-41. DOI: 10.4111/kju.2013.54.1.36. Epub 2013 Jan 18. Erratum in: Korean J Urol. 2013 Jun;54(6):415

[34] Parsons JK, Dahm P, Köhler TS, et al. Surgical management of lower urinary tract symptoms attributed to benign prostatic hyperplasia: AUA guideline amendment 2020. Journal of Urology. 2020;**204**:799

[35] Ito K, Takashima Y, Akamatsu S, Terada N, Kobayashi T, Yamasaki T, et al. Intravesical prostatic protrusion is not always the same shape: Evaluation by preoperative cystoscopy and outcome in HoLEP. Neurourology and Urodynamics. 2018;**37**(7):2160-2166. DOI: 10.1002/nau.23428. Epub 2018 Aug 10

[36] Bantis A, Zissimopoulos A, Kalaytzis C, Giannakopoulos S, Sountoulides P, Agelonidou E, et al. Correlation of serum prostate specific antigen, the volume and the intravesical prostatic protrusion for diagnosing bladder outlet obstruction in patients with benign prostate hyperplasia. Hellenic Journal of Nuclear Medicine. 2007;**10**(2):138-143. Greek, Modern. Erratum in: Hell J Nucl Med. 2010 Jan-Apr;13(1):78. Soundoulidis, Petros [corrected to Sountoulides, Petros]

[37] Rigatti L, Naspro R, Salonia A, Centemero A, Ghezzi M, Guazzoni G, et al. Urodynamics after TURP and HoLEP in urodynamically obstructed patients: Are there any differences at 1 year of follow-up? Urology. 2006;**67**(6):1193-1198. DOI: 10.1016/j.urology.2005.12.036

Chapter 3

Role of Endoscopic Retrograde Cholangiopancreatography in Benign Biliary Diseases

Lubna Kamani

Abstract

Endoscopic retrograde cholangiopancreatography (ERCP) is a combination of endoscopy and X-ray technique, which was introduced as a diagnostic tool but with the advancement in the technology such as balloon dilatation or stent placement in combination with ERCP has transformed the latter into therapeutic accessory for multiple biliary diseases. It can also be used as an adjunct tool to increase the success rate of therapy. This diversified application of ERCP emphasizes the importance of this procedure for patients with biliary diseases despite the certain post-interventional complications. The scope of ERCP procedure is continuously increasing in the detection of anatomical or physiological abnormalities. ERCP plays an important role in conditions with biliary obstruction or biliary leaks, which may be due to primary or secondary causes. Biliary stents can be placed in combination with ERCP, which can assist in achieving therapeutic goals in patients with biliary strictures or clearance of biliary sludge.

Keywords: endoscopic retrograde cholangiopancreatography, ERCP, benign biliary disease, choledocholithiasis, cholangitis

1. Introduction

Benign biliary diseases are diversified range of disorders, which may be congenital or acquired that can impact hepatic bile ducts and liver involvement. Incident diagnosis is very common in benign biliary diseases as the symptoms can vary from clinically asymptomatic to cholestatic symptoms with acute or chronic clinical path resulting in malignancy [1]. Patient workup is very important in determining the etiology of the disease, suggestive symptoms play a key role such as abdominal pain with fever can be due to choledocholithiasis, prior history of hepato-biliary surgery leading to biliary leak, autoimmune diseases, inflammatory strictures, and family history hereditary/congenital disorder [1].

Endoscopic retrograde cholangiopancreatography (ERCP), which uses combination of endoscopy and X-rays, was first introduced as a safe technique for diagnostic purpose of pancreaticobiliary disease. With the addition of endoscopic sphincterotomy technique, ERCP developed into therapeutic tool [2]. It is now considered to be gold standard for diagnosis of biliary-related diseases but also more reserved for

Benign Biliary diseases	
Cholelithiasis or gallstone disease	Choledocholithiasis
Post-surgical biliary complications	Bile leaks
	Biliary strictures
Stictures	Primary sclerosing cholangitis
	IgG4-related sclerosing cholangitis
	Ischemic cholangitis
	Inflammatory strictures
Developmental anomalies	Caroli's disease
	Choledochal cysts
Others	Sphincter of Oddi dysfunction
	Mirizzi Syndrome
	Parasites

Table 1.
Types of benign biliary disease.

therapeutic purpose owing to its more invasive nature when related to the alternative diagnostic tools [3]. Multiple imaging techniques are used in diagnosis for biliary disease such as intraoperative cholangiography, abdominal ultrasonography (US), computerized tomography (CT), magnetic resonance cholangiopancreatography (MRCP), and endoscopic ultrasound (EUS). They also play key role in determining the patient selection for ERCP to be considered as therapeutic intervention [4], but still the role of ERCP in differential diagnosis of multiple disease cannot be ruled out. ERCP can also be used in combination with other techniques such as cholangiopancreatoscopy where it applies as an adjunct for evaluation and management of biliary and pancreatic disease [5].

Endoscopists require extensive training to perform ERCP in order to increase the procedure success rate and also minimize as post-procedure complications such as bleeding, perforation, and pancreatitis which may lead to mortality and morbidity [6]. ERCP is precisely advantageous in the achievement of therapeutics in biliary obstructive patients due to choledocholithiasis, biliary leaks, or strictures where the success rates are found to be greater than 90% [7]. ERCP combined with bile duct stenting and/or biliary sphincterotomy is preferred when the diagnosis is bile leaks. Pre- and post-procedure antibiotic prophylaxis is recommended to all patients undergoing this procedure (**Table 1**).

2. Cholelithiasis or gallstone disease

Stone formation and presence in the biliary tree are referred to as cholelithiasis. This disease is one of the leading causes of hospital admissions worldwide and found to have prevalence rates of 3.2%–15.6% in Asia [8]. Stone location is the key to segmentation of this pathological condition as stones found in gall bladder and when the stones are located at extra hepatic bile ducts, it is referred to as choledocholithiasis, and intrahepatic stones presence causes hepatolithiasis. Stone formation is mainly due due to biliary stasis, which may be due to chemical imbalance of bile constituents or impaired gall bladder emptying. There are several risk factors for cholelithiasis, both modifiable and non-modifiable. Obesity is one of the major risk factors for cholilithiasis while other risk factors include dyslipidemias and insulin resistance Women are more prone to this pathological condition, whereas it has symmetrical relationship with the increase in age and is found to be asymptomatic in 80% of patients. Patients present with upper quadrant abdominal pain and positive for Murphy's sign. Abdominal ultrasound is found to be the most effective/noninvasive tool for diagnosis. The preferred treatment option for cholelithiasis is laproscopic cholecystectomy as an early intervention [9].

2.1 Choledocholithiasis

Choledocholithiasis is referred to a condition when stones are present in common bile duct (CBD). Exact prevalence is unknown, but studies have reported that about 5%–20% patients diagnosed with cholilithiasis have stones in CBD [10]. Choledocholithiasis may be classified into primary or secondary types where secondary refers to stones passage to bile ducts, and primary is due to conditions predisposing to bile stasis, which may be due to cystic fibrosis or long-term total parenteral nutrition. Choledocholithiasis might be due to complication of cholecystectomy procedure, which can be detected about after 3 years of surgery. Recurrent choledocholithiasis can also occur post cholecystectomy, which might be due to various secondary causes that include rapid weight loss (bariatric surgery), sickle cell anemia, periampullary duodenal diverticulum, chronic cholangitis, and dilated CBD or CBD stricture. Clinical features that distinguish choledocholithiasis are long-lasting post-prandial right upper quadrant (RUQ) pain that may exceed 6 hours, which may radiate to epigastrium or even back. Extrahepatic cholestatic signs may also be present, e.g., dark urine, pale stool, pruritis, etc. Evaluation should be done in all patients with or without presenting symptoms. First line of diagnostic tools are liver functioning tests (LFTs) and abdominal ultrasound. ERCP is the preferred diagnostic and therapeutic tool for confirming the likelihood of choledocholithiasis. ERCP has been reported to be very sensitive and specific in detection of CBD stones with the success rates of more than 95%, smaller stones may still be missed [11]. Air bubbles into biliary ductal system can lead to altered or misdiagnosis of stones; hence, introduction of air bubbles and over-filling of ducts by contrasts injections should be avoided. Characteristic findings for choledocholithiasis smooth-walled, well-defined, intraluminal defects within CBD, which may or may not be dilated. Management of choledocholithiasis initially includes support therapy for patients with acute symptoms with further identification of complications and management. Definitive treatment for choledocholithiasis is removal of CBD stone or elective cholecystectomy [10, 11]. In patients with no cholangitis or biliary obstruction, it is recommended to delay the ERCP procedure to >48 hours as it does not reduce the mortality rate when compared with conservative treatment [10]. However, it is reported that in patients with concomitant cholangitis with biliary obstruction, early ERCP reduces the mortality as well as adverse events following the procedure [12, 13]. Major complication that is found post ERCP is pancreatitis, which can increase the chances of mortality, which limits the use of ERCP in particular patients. This occurrence of complication like pancreatitis can be lowered with generous use of intravenous hydration and nonsteroidal anti-inflammatory rectal suppositories. For removal of larger stones, sphincterotomy combined with balloon sphincteroplasty and mechanical lithotripter can be used with high success of larger and difficult stone removal [14]. Moreover, where available, electrohydraulic lithotripsy may be used. However, if endoscopists failed to clear bile ducts, then plastic stent insertion is warranted for biliary drainage.

3. Post-surgical biliary complications

As the technological advancements and increase in use of laparoscopic techniques with shortened recovery times, decreased size of abdomen incision, it has become one of the first choices for treatment of biliary-related diseases. Concomitant use of laproscopic interventions has arisen a new complication of bile duct injury (BDI), which prevails in 0.2–1.4% of patients undergoing laparoscopic cholecystectomy [15, 16] and is reported to cause complications such as cystic duct leakage, CBD leakage, or bile duct strictures. Majority of post-surgical biliary complications can be treated successfully in 75–90% of patients by endoscopic or radiological interventions [17, 18].

3.1 Biliary leaks

Leakage of biliary constituents into abdominal cavity due to hole in bile duct, which may be due to postoperative complication. Biliary leaks can occur within a week of surgery but may present with symptoms even after a month of surgery. The symptoms present in the patient with such condition are nausea, vomiting, RUQ pain, jaundice, anorexia, and fever [19]. A distinct collection of bile outside biliary tree also known as biloma is a distinguished presentation of biliary leak, which can be encapsulated due to inflammatory reaction and fibrosis. Several imaging modalities can be applied for diagnosis of post-surgical biliary leaks or bilomas with abdominal ultrasound being the initial imaging took for quick and efficient follow-up for collection of biliary fluids [19]. Biloma can be present as ascitic fluid collection or well-confined loculated within particular boundaries, which is suggestive of an infection [20]. Computed tomography can also be used to detect bilomas and assess surrounding tissues where it can be used to study the further complications, e.g., biliary peritonitis. Source of biliary leakage can be identified by MRI and hepatobiliary cholescintigraphy [19]. Management of biliary leakage involves diversion and drainage of bilomas. Decompression of bile duct by sphincterotomy alone with or without endoscopic stent or nasobiliary drain placement. Stents are placed for 4–6 weeks, but larger duct injuries require longer duration of placement for healing of biliary leaks [21]. Biliary leaks can be segregated as low or high grade based on the extent of leakage after cholangiography, which can be identified during opacification. High-grade leaks are highly evident, whereas low grade requires complete filling of intrahepatic ducts to exhibit contrast extravasation. Location and grade of leak greatly influence the success rates of treatment with endoscopic procedure with range of 80–100% [22]. If ERCP and stenting fail, surgical correction is required.

3.2 Biliary strictures

Biliary strictures are a pathophysiological condition, which refers to constriction of intrahepatic or extrahepatic biliary ductal system. When this condition occurs, it hinders the normal flow of bile causing retention on bile and proximal dilatation, further causing biliary obstruction. Biliary strictures that are acquired are more common than congenital causes. Acquired biliary strictures are further classified into benign and malignant where 30% of biliary strictures are benign. During laparoscopic cholecystectomy, bile duct injury is due to misidentification of biliary duct for cystic duct that causes injury and clip application, which leads to formation of biliary strictures later on. Bile duct injury due to laparoscopic cholecystectomy accounts for 0.7% of total incidence of biliary strictures [23]. Recognition of blood supply is of prime importance for therapeutic procedures [24]. Anastomotic biliary strictures are complications arising from orthotopic liver transplantation or Whipple procedure (incidence rate is found to be 4%) performed for pancreatic mass or tumor [24, 25]. Biliary strictures can also be due to infections such as tuberculosis. However, the most common etiology for biliary strictures is malignancies [26]. Underlying etiology has shown to have strong impact on the prognosis of condition with strictures arising due to malignant, and primary sclerosing cholangitis may have unfavorable prognosis, whereas chronic pancreatitis, trauma, radiation, or operative injury has a good prognosis. Strictures identified in an early stage respond better to endoscopic treatment, which involves serial placement of single or multiple plastic stents over a period of 1 year. Fully covered metal stents are available for benign strictures and can be removed later [27, 28]. Success rates for this procedure range from 74 to 90% but have a very high recurrence rate after the removal of stents, a more aggressive approach is found to have more consistent results. Late anastomotic strictures require long term and multiple therapies (1–2 years). Balloon dilation is found to be less effective than combination of balloon dilation and stent placement, which has response rates of 70–100%. Subsequently increment in the number of stents post ERCP is reported to be most effective therapeutic approach [29]. Post-surgical biliary-enteric anastomosis can be treated successfully with ERCP, which might be assisted with enteroscopy for stricture site access.

4. Sclerosing cholangitis

Sclerosing cholangitis is spectrum of pathological condition, which encompasses the inflammation of intrahepatic and/or extrahepatic bile ducts, which is progressive. Fibrosis, stricturing, and patchy inflammation are characteristic presentation of sclerosing cholangitis. The course of diseases varies greatly in involvement of bile ducts complicated by carcinoma even at early stages of disease or subtle occurrence of portal hypertension leading to cirrhosis and hepatic failure [30]. Sclerosing cholangitis can be differentiated into different types based on causative agents or factors ranging from unknown to known factors such as infections, pancreatic disorders, etc.

4.1 Primary sclerosing cholangitis

Primary sclerosing cholangitis (PSC) is the most common form of cholangitis. Exact etiology is unknown, but some of the literatures associate this with autoimmune conditions such as ulcerative colitis (UC). Inflammatory bowel disease accompanies PSC in 90% of patients, where 87% of patients have comorbidity with either Crohn's disease or ulcerative colitis. However, approximately 5% of UC and $\leq 5\%$ of Crohn's disease develop PSC. Cholangitis is initially asymptomatic, which after progression shows signs of cholestasis and in the later stages may transform to cirrhosis. Males are more prone to this condition in comparison to females [31, 32]. Approach for diagnostics should be focused on the laboratory reports and radiological tests where persistent elevated cholestatic enzymes are sign of presence of PSC. Biliary obstruction is corrected with ERCP to clear stenosis. Multiple stenting might be required for certain patients. ERCP is discouraged in the diagnosis of PSC due to its possibility of adverse events such as bacterial cholangitis, perforation of biliary tract, and pancreatitis. However, diagnostic use of ERCP in PSC has proven to be advantageous in certain conditions. It may facilitate the diagnosis of PSC, which is not determined by magnetic resonance cholangiopancreatography due to suboptimal imaging of intrahepatic bile ducts [33]. Secondly, it can also determine the prevailing stricture with high accuracy in patients with deteriorating conditions, which may present as persisting cholestasis, jaundice, or bacterial cholangitis. ERCP can also precisely establish existing cholangiocarcinoma, which can be misidentified for biliary stricture that possesses symptoms of biliary dilatation [33]. Strictures that are associated with PSC have positive prognosis with endoscopic intervention such as balloon dilation, which can be accompanied by stent placement. Since there are high chances of adverse reactions or complications, balloon dilatation is found to be sufficient, but the literature data are limited. Therefore, stent placement is preferred for dominant strictures, which are unmanageable by dilatation leading to increase in the chances of survival of patients with PSC.

4.2 IgG4-related sclerosing cholangitis

IgG4-related sclerosing cholangitis (IgG-SC) is a fibro-inflammatory disease with systemic involvement with classical findings for lesions and fibrosis in the biliary system. IgG-SC may have symptoms similar as PSC or pancreatic adenocarcinoma. Pathology of the condition varies from inflammatory stage to fibrosis to organ failure and even mortality. Epidemiological data for IgG-SC are very limited. IgG-SC is predominantly found in males usually affecting in fifth and sixth decade of life [34]. Epidemiological studies report chronic exposure to "blue collar work" to be associated with incidence of IgG-SC [35, 36]. Clinical history for chronic allergy with elevated levels of IgE directly correlates with the occurrence of IgG-SC. Clinical presentation for IgG-SC depends on the organ involved and the extent of disease. IgG-SC can affect any part of biliary tree. Obstructive jaundice, weight loss, and RUQ abdominal pain are associated with the presence of IgG-SC. Patients with IgG-SC can be spontaneously identified by abnormal liver functioning test and elevated markers for inflammation. Total IgG concentrations may or may not be elevated despite IgG-4 subclass concentrations being elevated [33]. ERCP alone as a diagnostic tool for IgG-SC has low level of accuracy to differentiate between IgG-SC and PSC or cholangiocarcinoma where cross-sectional imaging plays an important role in identification of IgG-SC. ERCP and biliary stenting help in symptomatic relief.

4.3 Ischemic cholangitis

Injury to any vessel or vessels supplying blood to biliary tract can causing impaired blood supply, which can be focal or extensive depending on the extent of injury. Formation of lesions in biliary system due to restricted blood flow is labelled as ischemic cholangitis (IC) [37]. Blood flow restriction that can cause IC can be at the level of major hepatic arteries or at microvascular plexus level. Damage to the vessels during liver transplantation or radiation therapy is among few of the common causes of IC. Hypercoagulative disorders can also cause thrombosis resulting in IC. The underlying factors related to ischemic biliary damage are arduous to identify as it has high mortality rate [38]. Lesions due to IC can be subdivided into extrahepatic and intrahepatic lesions or combination of both due to success rates of therapy. IC may be asymptomatic in the initial stage with majority of IC showing signs post 6 months to a year of post-surgical intervention, with rarely secluded extrahepatic or intrahepatic involvement. Major presenting signs of IC are cholangitis and cholestasis, which are aggressively progressive leading to hepatocellular failure. Ischemic injury is prominent factor for recurrent signs of cholangitis. IC is not reversible, and management options are very limited. Uncomplicated IC is not associated with high risk of mortality but is likely to have high morbidity due to extensive invasive procedures of multiple dilatations and hospitalizations. Diffused IC requires ERCP with stricture dilatation and stent placement. Application of percutaneous transhepatic cholangiography-guided drainage if ERCP fails or hepaticojejunostomy may be required in conditions that are difficult to manage [39]. Endoscopic therapy is considered to be first line of IC strictures and is minimally invasive; it can also play an adjuvant role in bridging during liver retransplantation. Process of ERCP dwells removal of biliary sludge and casts. Since biliary strictures in IC are bilobar, diffused, and accompany high predilection for intrahepatic ducts, insertion of stent post balloon dilation is required [40]. Patients with IC may require stent replacement every 3–4 months [41].

4.4 Recurrent pyogenic cholangitis

Biliary tree can be infested by parasitic organisms causing inflammatory disease leading to scarring of bile duct tissue ultimately followed by bile stasis, intrahepatic stones, stricture formation, and even portal hypertension. This condition is also known as pyogenic cholangitis, since it is associated with recurrent attacks; it is referred to as recurrent pyogenic cholangitis (RPC) [42, 43]. Hepatolithiasis can also cause RPC, which further leads to recurrent bacterial infections and biliary inflammation. It is also known as oriental cholangiohepatitis, exact etiology is unknown, but some literature reports association with *Ascaris lumbricoides and Clonorchis sinensis.* The involvement of parasites is unclear in the etiology of RPC, where data suggest debilitation of immunity allowing bacterial infestations, scarring, and fibrosis and ultimate stricture formation. Epidemiological data report RPC to be prevalent in Asian population, but it can also be found in American regions. Recently, the incidence rate of this disease is found to be in declining phase due to increment in the habitat standards and Westernization of diet. Therefore, demographic details play an important role in diagnosis of the disease. Common laboratory findings report elevated leucocyte count and levels of bilirubin. Patient suffering from RPC shows a much diversified range of symptoms, mild symptoms to fulminant abdominal sepsis. Radiological techniques are further used for confirmation of presence of RPC. Previously, direct cholangiography was considered to be first line, but ERCP has shown certain advantage over the former where extrahepatic strictures can be well identified using ERCP, and it permits better evaluation of peripheral ducts due to better spatial resolution. It provides both evaluation for diagnosis and therapeutic intervention in a single procedure. The aim of therapy is to achieve unobstructed flow of bile by eliminating calculi from biliary tree and prevention of further stone formation. In patients with extractable stones ERCP technique, which is reported to effective in 90% of the cases [42, 43]. Balloon angioplasty catheters can also be used for stricture dilatation, and plastic stents may be inserted to ensure integrity of decompressed duct. Fully covered metal stents can also be used because of their long term patency; however, because of benign nature of disease and high cost of metal stent, therefore, it is not recommended to use metal stents in this condition [44].

5. Developmental anomalies

Pancreaticobiliary tree developmental anomalies may remain until later stages of adolescence or early adulthood. Unexplained signs and recurrent symptoms related to biliary tree issues such as abdominal pain, jaundice, nausea, and vomiting should trigger the presence of congenital anomaly and cholangiopancreatography should be warranted. Detection of developmental anomalies may facilitate in therapeutics and prevention of ductal injury. Developmental anomalies of biliary tree include Caroli's disease, choledochal cysts, and Von Meyenburg complexes.

5.1 Caroli's disease

Caroli's disease (CD) is congenital anomaly of intrahepatic bile ducts accustomed by segmented cystic dilation of ducts. It is reported to develop from abnormal ductal plate malformation during developmental phase of biliary tree. It is theoretically explained to follow autosomal dominant inheritance in some families. CD can remain unnoticed during the first stages of life and can also remain the same for whole life. Dominant symptoms are progressive recurrent cholangitis, intrahepatic calculi, and abscesses and may also lead to sepsis. Liver transplantation is the definite treatment and required in some cases [45]. Males and females are equally prone to this condition with 80% of the cases being identified before the age of 30 [46, 47]. ERCP is reported to be very highly sensitive for diagnosis of CD perhaps some of the literature reports it to be of highest sensitivity [48]. Saccular dilatation is the distinguishing sign that confirms the presence of CD as the symptoms can be misidentified for PSC or RPC. Due to the distinguishing feature, identification of cystic lesions across the biliary tree is an important factor in diagnosis, which is accurately accomplished by ERCP. Positive evaluation of transient recovery from cholangitis by ERCP also gives an additional benefit of utilizing ERCP procedure in CD.

5.2 Choledocal cysts

Choledocal cyst (CC) is one of the benign anomalies of congenital origin, which is associated with dilatation of intrahepatic or extrahepatic bile ducts. Approximately 1% of benign biliary diseases are CC [49]. It has high prevalence in Asian population with predominance in females. The incidence literature is very scarce with few studies reporting to be one in 13,000–2,000,000 live births. CC can be diagnosed in any part of life, but approximately 50% of the cases are diagnosed in the first decade of life. Many hypotheses have been proposed regarding origin of CC but the widely accepted is the association with abnormality in the arrangement of pancreaticobiliary ductal junction during development [49]. The pancreatio-cobiliary junction is situated near to the sphincter of Oddi, this common pathway causes retrograde flux of pancreatic juice into biliary tree causing inflammation, ectasia, and dilatation. Clinical presentation includes classic biliary symptoms in adults and with abdominal mass as distinguishing feature for CC in infants. But, this abdominal mass is physically palpable in approximately up to 60% of cases [50, 51]; therefore, diagnosis of CC cannot be ruled out in the absence. CC is segregated in different types according to the involvement of portion of biliary tree. The most common complication of CC is stone formation and malignancy. ERCP is considered to be gold standard for diagnosis of CC as it is found to be safe of patients of all ages. ERCP can play therapeutic role in CC where biliary obstruction is found, whereas it is equally effective in giving clear picture of ductal anatomy for prior strategizing for definite surgical intervention. ERCP not only is effective in preoperative phase, but it can play important role in post-surgical phase in clearance of biliary sludge and monitoring of integrity of biliary tree [50, 52].

6. Others

6.1 Sphincter of Oddi dysfunction

Sphincter of Oddi (SD) is a muscular valve situated in the duodenum, which regulates the flow of pancreatic or hepatic contents into the small intestine. Prevention of accumulation of bile sludge and particulate matter is one of the distinguished functions, thus reducing the probability of inflammation. Failure to perform this function is known as sphincter of Oddi dysfunction (SOD). Prevalence of SOD is found to be 1.5% in general population, which increases to 23% in patients showing signs of biliary disease [53, 54]. SOD may occur in adult or pediatric population, but it is found to be more prevalent in middle-aged women [54]. SOD might relate to a prior cholecystectomy, which changes the dynamics of biliary system. Symptoms of SOD and gall bladder dysfunction cannot be distinguished; therefore, proper investigations are required to diagnose SOD. Classic biliary disease symptoms are also found in SOD, presence of which is the basis of classification of SOD. There are multiple diagnostic (invasive and noninvasive) methods that can be useful in identifying SOD, but gold standard is the use of Sphincter of Oddi manometry (SOM), which observes the motor activity of SD with the use of ERCP technique [55]. Despite technical hassle and expertise, SOM is widely accepted and used for diagnosis of SOD. SOM is indicated in patients with unexplained excruciating pancreatobiliary pain with or without abnormal liver enzymes. Some literature reports also suggest that SOM can also predict the outcome of sphincter ablation in the SOD patients [56]. The therapy for SOD is evolving with major aim to establish reflow of biliary or pancreatic content to intestine. Since there is very limited evidence of medical therapy, traditionally surgical therapy was preferred choice However, use of less invasive laparoscopic techniques is preferred. Transduodenal biliary sphincterplasty with pancreatic septoplasty is the most common surgical intervention but due to patient tolerance, cost of care, morbidity, and mortality, this approach is being minimized. At present, surgical intervention is only reserved for patients who have undergone through endoscopic procedure previously and symptoms have reemerged or if the endoscopic procedure is not feasible [56]. However, for pancreatic sphincter hypertension, surgical intervention is considered to be standard of care [57]. ERCP is termed as standard for type I and II SOD as it responds with positive etiology to ERCP [58]. Endoscopic sphincterotomy related to sphincter ablation is reported to have clinical improvement in about 90% of patients with SOD. Pancreatic sphincter hypertension is related to the failure of endoscopic interventions in patients as pancreatic sphincter pressure is unaltered even when biliary sphincter pressure is compressed [59]. Balloon dilatation and stent placements, which can become very common in GI strictures, are not currently known to be useful in SOD due to limited evidence [56]. Literature data are suggestive that ERCP along with manometric evaluations is the current standard for diagnosis and predictive of further therapy associated with SOD.

6.2 Mirizzi syndrome

Mirrizzi syndrome (MS) is complication of long-term cholilithiasis, with the prevalence of 0.05–2.7% among high-risk patients with calculus of gallbladder [60, 61]. MS is the presence of gall stones in gall bladder or cystic ducts that causes extrinsic compression of common hepatic duct. Due to compression of ducts, the process of inflammation is initiated. Chronic inflammation leads gall bladder to shrink and partially fused with hepatic duct. Impaction of gall stone and shrunken gall bladder results in stricture and pressure necrosis of intervening wall, ultimately fistula formation [62, 63]. Clinical presentation for MS is features of obstructive jaundice and abdominal pain with or without any pathognomonic features on history and physical examination. Classification of MS is based on ERCP finding according to the positioning, presence of stone and fistula. Females are more prone to MS in comparison to males. This gender affinity toward females is associated with the higher incidence of gall stones in female gender [64]. Diagnosis in the earlier stages of MS is very significant as unidentified MS may result in biliary duct injuries as a consequence [65]. Currently, ERCP is gold standard for diagnosing MS as it also gives information regarding the cause and extent of biliary obstruction and the damage to the ducts. ERCP also distinguishes ductal abnormalities including presence of fistulas [66, 67]. Percutaneous transhepatic cholangiography (PTC) can also be used for diagnosis of MS, but it has less efficiency than ERCP, which can identify a low lying stone in cystic duct that is often missed by PTC. Furthermore, visualization of distal common biliary duct is hindered if there is obstruction at any level of common hepatic duct, whereas ERCP can also be used as therapeutic procedure for MS. Open surgical management is the standard of therapy in MS with positive results reported and decrease in overall mortality and morbidity [68]. Endoscopic procedures with therapeutic goal are reserved for patients who are poor candidate for surgery (e.g., elderly with multiple comorbidities) where stent placement can achieve the patency of common hepatic duct [69].

6.3 Biliary worms

Parasitic infections are common in biliary tree, which are due to manifestations of nematodes and hermaphroditic trematodes. These parasitic infestations may cause diversified pathologies ranging from cholithiasis to pancreatitis to liver abscess [70]. Presence of worms in stools and duodenal contents confirms the diagnosis of biliary infestation. ERCP is a very useful tool not only in diagnosis but also aims for removal of biliary worms. More than 80% of patients with biliary ascariasis are treated successfully by ERCP [71]. Treatment of ascariasis may or may not require sphincterotomy and balloon dilation. Both of which can be performed in a single session of ERCP setting. Children are more prone to parasitic infestations, and ERCP is also found to be safe and effective for this population as well.

7. Conclusion

Endoscopic procedures are now preferred over surgical interventions due to less invasive in nature, cost of therapy, and patient compliance. ERCP plays an important role in diagnosis and therapeutics of multiple benign biliary diseases. Despite risk of post-procedural complications such as pancreatitis, bleeding, or perforation, it is considered to be one of the most effective tools with or without combination of interventions such as balloon dilation or stent placements. ERCP can also play a transitional role in biliary surgery as a temporary intervention to further strategize the therapeutics of biliary diseases.

Author details

Lubna Kamani
Liaquat National Hospital, Karachi, Pakistan

*Address all correspondence to: lkamani@yahoo.com

References

[1] European Association for the Study of the Liver. EASL Clinical Practice Guidelines: Management of cholestatic liver diseases. Journal of Hepatology. 2009;**51**(2):237-267

[2] McCune WS, Shorb PE, Moscovitz H. Endoscopic cannulation of the ampulla of vater: A preliminary report. Annals of Surgery. 1968;**167**(5):752

[3] Bali MA, Pezzullo M, Pace E, Morone M. Benign biliary diseases. European Journal of Radiology. 2017;**93**:217-228

[4] NIH Consensus Development Program. NIH state-of-the-science statement on endoscopic retrograde cholangiopancreatography (ERCP) for diagnosis and therapy. National Institutes of Health, Office of the Director. Indiana University; 2002

[5] Chathadi KV, Chandrasekhara V, Acosta RD, Decker GA, Early DS, Eloubeidi MA, et al. The role of ERCP in benign diseases of the biliary tract. Gastrointestinal Endoscopy. 2015;**81**(4):795-803

[6] Chandrasekhara V, Khashab MA, Muthusamy VR, Acosta RD, Agrawal D, Bruining DH, et al. Adverse events associated with ERCP. Gastrointestinal Endoscopy. 2017;**85**(1):32-47

[7] Costamagna G, Shah SK, Tringali A. Current management of postoperative complications and benign biliary strictures. Gastrointestinal Endoscopy Clinics. 2003;**13**(4):635-648

[8] Gyedu A, Adae-Aboagye K, Badu-PeprahA.Prevalenceofcholelithiasis among persons undergoing abdominal ultrasound at the Komfo Anokye Teaching Hospital, Kumasi, Ghana. African Health Sciences. 2015;**15**(1):246-252

[9] European Association for the Study of the Liver. EASL Clinical Practice Guidelines on the prevention, diagnosis and treatment of gallstones. Journal of Hepatology. 2016;**65**:146-181

[10] Buxbaum JL, Fehmi SM, Sultan S, Fishman DS, Qumseya BJ, Cortessis VK, et al. ASGE guideline on the role of endoscopy in the evaluation and management of choledocholithiasis. Gastrointestinal Endoscopy. 2019;**89**(6):1075-1105

[11] Williams EJ, Green J, Beckingham I, Parks R, Martin D, Lombard M. Guidelines on the management of common bile duct stones (CBDS). Gut. 1 Jul 2008;**57**(7):1004-1021

[12] Tse F, Yuan Y. Early Routine Endoscopic Retrograde Cholangiopancreatography (ERCP) Strategy versus Early Conservative Management Strategy in Acute Gallstone Pancreatitis: A Cochrane Systematic Review and Meta-analysis Presidential Poster: 157. Official journal of the American College of Gastroenterology| ACG. 1 Oct 2012;107:S67

[13] Maple JT, Ben-Menachem T, Anderson MA, Appalaneni V, Banerjee S, Cash BD, et al. The role of endoscopy in the evaluation of suspected choledocholithiasis. Gastrointestinal Endoscopy. 2010;**7**(1):1-9

[14] Meine GC, Baron TH. Endoscopic papillary large-balloon dilation combined with endoscopic biliary sphincterotomy for the removal of bile duct stones (with video). Gastrointestinal Endoscopy. 2011;**74**(5):1119-1126

[15] Giger UF, Michel JM, Opitz I, Inderbitzin DT, Kocher T, Krähenbühl L, et al. Risk factors for perioperative complications in patients undergoing laparoscopic cholecystectomy: Analysis of 22,953 consecutive cases from the swiss Association of Laparoscopic and Thoracoscopic Surgery database. Journal of the American College of Surgeons. 2006;**203**(5):723-728

[16] Richardson MC, Bell G, Fullarton GM. Incidence and nature of bile duct injuries following laparoscopic cholecystectomy: An audit of 5913 cases. West of Scotland laparoscopic cholecystectomy audit group. British Journal of Surgery. 1996;**83**(10):1356-1360

[17] De Reuver PR, Busch OR, Rauws EA, Lameris JS, Van Gulik TM, Gouma D. Long-term results of a primary end-to-end anastomosis in peroperative detected bile duct injury. Journal of Gastrointestinal Surgery. 2007;**11**(3):296-302

[18] Rauws EA, Gouma DJ. Endoscopic and surgical management of bile duct injury after laparoscopic cholecystectomy. Best Practice & Research. Clinical Gastroenterology. 2004;**18**(5):829-846

[19] Nikpour AM, Knebel RJ, Cheng D. Diagnosis and Management of Postoperative Biliary Leaks. Seminars in Interventional Radiology. Dec 2016;**33**(4):307-312. DOI: 10.1055/s-0036-1592324. PMID: 27904250; PMCID: PMC5088090

[20] Copelan A, Bahoura L, Tardy F, Kirsch M, Sokhandon F, Kapoor B. Etiology, diagnosis, and management of bilomas: a current update. Techniques in vascular and interventional radiology. 1 Dec 2015;**18**(4):236-243

[21] Seeras K, Qasawa RN, Kashyap S, et al. Bile Duct Repair. [Updated 2022 Jun 5]. In: StatPearls [Internet]. Treasure Island, FL: StatPearls Publishing; 2022. Available from: https://www.ncbi.nlm.nih.gov/books/NBK525989/

[22] Shanbhogue AK, Tirumani SH, Prasad SR, Fasih N, McInnes M. Benign biliary strictures: A current comprehensive clinical and imaging review. American Journal of Roentgenology. 2011;**197**(2):W295-W306

[23] Paranandi B, Oppong KW. Biliary strictures: Endoscopic assessment and management. Frontline Gastroenterology. 2017;**8**(2):133-137

[24] Costamagna G, Pandolfi M, Mutignani M, Spada C, Perri V. Long-term results of endoscopic management of postoperative bile duct strictures with increasing numbers of stents. Gastrointestinal Endoscopy. 2001;**54**(2):162-168

[25] Kassab C, Prat F, Liguory C, Meduri B, Ducot B, Fritsch J, et al. Endoscopic management of post-laparoscopic cholecystectomy biliary strictures: Long-term outcome in a multicenter study. Gastroentérologie Clinique et Biologique. 2006;**30**(1):124-129

[26] Zepeda-Gómez S, Baron TH. Benign biliary strictures: Current endoscopic management. Nature Reviews. Gastroenterology & Hepatology. 2011;**8**(10):573-581

[27] Feldman M, Friedman L, Sleisenger M. Sleisenger & Fordtran's Gastro-Intestinal and Liver Disease: Pathophysiology, Diagnosis and Manage-Ment. 7th ed. Philadelphia: Saunders; 2002. pp. 1131-1137

[28] Kowdley KV. Primary Sclerosing Cholangitis: Epidemiology and Pathogenesis. Waltham, MA; 2015

[29] Primary Sclerosing Cholangitis. 2022. Available from: https://next.amboss.com/us/article/nS07Zf?q=Sclerosing%20cholangitis#Z17ab40a6a2ee805421ace9478cfb909c [Accessed: August 26, 2022]

[30] Baluyut AR, Sherman S, Lehman GA, Hoen H, Chalasani N. Impact of endoscopic therapy on the survival of patients with primary sclerosing cholangitis. Gastrointestinal Endoscopy. 2001;**53**(3):308-312

[31] Singh S, Talwalkar JA. Primary sclerosing cholangitis: Diagnosis, prognosis, and management. Clinical Gastroenterology and Hepatology. 2013;**11**(8):898-907

[32] Ghazale A, Chari ST, Zhang L, Smyrk TC, Takahashi N, Levy MJ, et al. Immunoglobulin G4–associated cholangitis: Clinical profile and response to therapy. Gastroenterology. 2008;**134**(3):706-715

[33] Culver EL, Webster G. IgG4-related sclerosing cholangitis. Biliary Disease. 2017:243-261

[34] Skaro AI, Jay CL, Baker TB, Wang E, Pasricha S, Lyuksemburg V, et al. The impact of ischemic cholangiopathy in liver transplantation using donors after cardiac death: The untold story. Surgery. 2009;**146**(4):543

[35] de Buy Wenniger LJ, Culver EL, Beuers U. Exposure to occupational antigens might predispose to IgG4-related disease. Hepatology (Baltimore, Md.). 2014;**60**(4):1453

[36] Campbell WL, Sheng R, Zajko AB, Abu-Elmagd K, Demetris AJ. Intrahepatic biliary strictures after liver transplantation. Radiology. 1994;**191**(3):735-740

[37] Tung BY, Kimmey MB. Biliary complications of orthotopic liver transplantation. Digestive Diseases. 1999;**17**(3):133-144

[38] Guichelaar MM, Benson JT, Malinchoc M, Krom RA, Wiesner RH, Charlton MR. Risk factors for and clinical course of non-anastomotic biliary strictures after liver transplantation. American Journal of Transplantation. 2003;**3**(7):885-890

[39] Okuno WT, Whitman GJ, Chew FS. Recurrent pyogenic cholangiohepatitis. American journal of roentgenology. 1996;**167**(2):484

[40] Afagh A, Pancu D. Radiologic findings in recurrent pyogenic cholangitis. The Journal of Emergency Medicine. 2004;**26**(3):343-346

[41] Gupta A, Simo K. Recurrent Pyogenic Cholangitis. In: StatPearls [Internet]. Treasure Island, FL: StatPearls Publishing; 9 May 2022. PMID: 33231978

[42] Jain M, Agarwal A. MRCP findings in recurrent pyogenic cholangitis. European Journal of Radiology. 2008;**66**(1):79-83

[43] Al-Sukhni W, Gallinger S, Pratzer A, Wei A, Ho CS, Kortan P, et al. Recurrent pyogenic cholangitis with hepatolithiasis—The role of surgical therapy in North America. Journal of Gastrointestinal Surgery. 2008;**12**(3):496-503

[44] Yoon HK, Sung KB, Song HY, Kang SG, Kim MH, Lee SG, et al. Benign biliary strictures associated with recurrent pyogenic cholangitis: Treatment with expandable metallic stents. American Journal of Roentgenology. 1997;**169**(6):1523-1527

[45] Waechter FL, Sampaio JA, Pinto RD, Alvares-da-Silva MR, Cardoso FG,

Francisconi C, et al. The role of liver transplantation in patients with Caroli's disease. Hepato-Gastroenterology. 2001;**48**(39):672-674

[46] Lu SC, Debian KA. Cystic diseases of the biliary tract. In: Yamada T, Alpers DH, Kaplowitz N, Laine L, Owyang C, Powell DW, editors. Textbook of Gastroenterology. Philadelphia: Lippincott Williams and Wilkins; 2003. pp. 2225-2233

[47] Yonem O, Bayraktar Y. Clinical characteristics of Caroli's disease. World Journal of Gastroenterology. 2007;**13**(13):1930

[48] Saxena R, Pradeep R, Chander J, Kumar P, Wig JD, Yadav RV, et al. Benign disease of the common bile duct. The British Journal of Surgery. 1988;**75**(8):803-806

[49] Olbourne NA, Choledochal cysts. A review of the cystic anomalies of the biliary tree. Annals of the Royal College of Surgeons of England. 1975;**56**(1):26

[50] Tan SS, Tan NC, Ibrahim S, Tay KH. Management of adult choledochal cyst. Singapore Medical Journal. 2007;**48**(6):524

[51] Choledochal Cyst. 2022. Available from: https://radiopaedia.org/articles/choledochal-cyst. [Accessed August 28, 2022]

[52] De Angelis P, Foschia F, Romeo E, Caldaro T, Rea F, Di Abriola GF, et al. Role of endoscopic retrograde cholangiopancreatography in diagnosis and management of congenital choledochal cysts: 28 pediatric cases. Journal of Pediatric Surgery. 2012;**47**(5):885-888

[53] Drossman DA, Li Z, Andruzzi E, Temple RD, Talley NJ, Grant Thompson W, et al. US householder survey of functional gastrointestinal disorders. Digestive Diseases and Sciences. 1993;**38**(9):1569-1580

[54] Corazziari E, Shaffer EA, Hogan WJ, Sherman S, Toouli J. Functional disorders of the biliary tract and pancreas. Gut. 1999;**45**(2):48-54

[55] Cheon YK. How to interpret a functional or motility test-sphincter of oddi manometry. Journal of Neurogastroenterology and Motility. 2012;**18**(2):211

[56] Sherman S. What is the role of ERCP in the setting of abdominal pain of pancreatic or biliary origin (suspected sphincter of Oddi dysfunction)? Gastrointestinal Endoscopy. 2002;**56**(6):S258-S266

[57] Kuo WH, Pasricha PJ, Kalloo AN. The role of sphincter of Oddi manometry in the diagnosis and therapy of pancreatic disease. Gastrointestinal Endoscopy Clinics of North America. 1998;**8**(1):79-85

[58] Lim CH, Jahansouz C, Freeman ML, Leslie DB, Ikramuddin S, Amateau SK. Outcomes of endoscopic retrograde cholangiopancreatography (ERCP) and sphincterotomy for suspected sphincter of Oddi dysfunction (SOD) post Roux-en-Y gastric bypass. Obesity Surgery. 2017;**27**(10):2656-2662

[59] Sherman S, Hawes RH, Madura JA, Lehman GA. Comparison of intraoperative and endoscopic manometry of the sphincter of Oddi. Surgery, Gynecology & Obstetrics. 1992;**175**(5):410-418

[60] Abou-Saif A, Al-Kawas FH. Complications of gallstone disease: Mirizzi syndrome, cholecystocholedochal fistula, and

gallstone ileus. The American journal of gastroenterology. 2002;**97**(2):249-254

[61] Curet MJ, Rosendale DE, Congilosi S. Mirizzi syndrome in a native American population. The American journal of surgery. 1994;**168**(6):616-621

[62] Tanaka N, Nobori M, Furuya T, Ueno T, Kimura H, Nagai M, et al. Evolution of Mirizzi syndrome with biliobiliary fistula. Journal of Gastroenterology. 1995;**30**(1):117-121

[63] Csendes A, Diaz JC, Burdiles P, Maluenda F, Nava O. Mirizzi syndrome and cholecystobiliary fistula: A unifying classification. Journal of British Surgery. 1989;**76**(11):1139-1143

[64] Ahlawat SK, Singhania R, Al-Kawas FH. Mirizzi syndrome. Current Treatment Options in Gastroenterology. 2007;**10**(2):102-110

[65] Tan KY, Chng HC, Chen CY, Tan SM, Poh BK, Hoe MN. Mirizzi syndrome: Noteworthy aspects of a retrospective study in one Centre. ANZ Journal of Surgery. 2004;**74**(10):833-837

[66] Cruz FO, Barriga P, Tocornal J, Burhenne HJ. Radiology of the Mirizzi syndrome: Diagnostic importance of the transhepatic cholangiogram. Gastrointestinal Radiology. 1983;**8**(1):249-253

[67] Ravo B, Epstein H, La Mendola S, Ger R. The Mirizzi syndrome: Preoperative diagnosis by sonography and transhepatic cholangiography. American Journal of Gastroenterology (Springer Nature). 1986;**81**(8)

[68] Khan TF, Muniandy S, Hayat FZ, Sherazi ZA, Nawaz MH. Mirizzi syndrome--a report of 3 cases with a review of the present classifications. Singapore Medical Journal. 1999;**40**(3):171-173

[69] Chowbey PK, Sharma A, Mann V, Khullar R, Baijal M, Vashistha A. The management of Mirizzi syndrome in the laparoscopic era. Surgical Laparoscopy, Endoscopy & Percutaneous Techniques. 2000;**10**(1):11-14

[70] Bektaş M, Dökmeci A, Cinar K, Halici I, Oztas E, Karayalcin S, et al. Endoscopic management of biliary parasitic diseases. Digestive Diseases and Sciences. 2010;**55**(5):1472-1478

[71] Sandouk F, Haffar S, Zada MM, Graham DY, Anand BS. Pancreatic-biliary ascariasis: Experience of 300 cases. American Journal of Gastroenterology (Springer Nature). 1997;**92**(12)

Chapter 4

SLAP Lesions in Overhead Athletes

William B. Stetson, Katie Lutz and Kristen Reikersdorfer

Abstract

Superior labral anterior to posterior (SLAP) tears in overhead athletes can be a career-ending injury because of the high failure rates with surgical intervention. There are many factors for this including the failure to establish the correct diagnosis, inadequate nonoperative management, the repair of normal variants of the superior labrum by inexperienced surgeons, and improper poor surgical technique. SLAP lesions rarely occur in isolation and can be associated with other shoulder disorders. The mechanism of injury can be an acute episode of trauma or a history of repetitive overhead use as in baseball pitchers or volleyball players. The physical exam findings can be confusing as these injuries often occur with other shoulder pathology. There is no single physical exam finding that is pathognomonic for SLAP tears. Nonoperative treatment should always be undertaken for a minimum of 3 months before surgery is recommended. If this fails to return the overhead athlete to competitive participation, a diagnostic arthroscopy with SLAP repair can yield excellent results if the proper technique is employed. The technique that we describe can be technically demanding but can be reproduced and give excellent results with a predictable return to play for overhead athletes.

Keywords: SLAP tears, overhead athletes, shoulder, arthroscopy

1. Introduction

Superior labral tears anterior to posterior, the so-called SLAP lesion, coined by Snyder and colleagues, are a common injury in overhead athletes. Snyder described four different types of SLAP lesions and found that they were uncommon [1]. In a retrospective review of more than 700 shoulder arthroscopies at the Southern California Orthopedic Institute (SCOI), Snyder et al. identified 27 patients who had significant pathology of the superior labrum at the time of arthroscopy [1]. Although SLAP tears can be rare, they can be a source of significant disability [1, 2]. Andrews, Carson and McLeod [3] first reported on a group of athletes who had tears of the anterosuperior labrum not extending posterior to the biceps. The authors felt that this injury pattern was due to repetitive traction of the biceps on the labrum as a result of repeated throwing motions.

The Snyder classification system presents an organized approach to defining SLAP pathology, the challenge is to diagnose these lesions properly and to differentiate significant superior labral pathology from the many normal anatomic variations that exist [4].

With the advent of shoulder arthroscopy in the late 1980s and early 1990s, it became possible to diagnose these injury patterns, which were difficult to diagnose with radiographic methods at that time. Shoulder arthroscopy has helped delineate specific injury patterns of the superior labrum [5].

The SLAP lesion injury pattern involves the superior aspect of the glenoid labrum in which the tear begins posteriorly and extends anteriorly, stopping at or above the mid-glenoid notch. The superior labrum is functionally important as it serves as the “anchor” for the insertion of the long head of the biceps tendon [1]. Injuries to the biceps tendon attachment to the superior glenoid labrum can be acute or chronic.

The incidence of SLAP tears varies. Maffet et al. [6] reported 84 of 712 patients or a 12% incidence of SLAP tears, whereas Handelberg et al. [7] reported a 6% incidence (32 of 530 patients). Snyder and colleagues [1] reported a 4% incidence of SLAP tears in their original description in 1990.

The etiology of SLAP lesions remains uncertain, but there are many theories on its pathogenesis including acute trauma or repetitive overhead activities.

SLAP lesions have been identified in association with shoulder instability but can occur in association with diagnoses other than instability [1, 6–9]. The difficulty lies in the preoperative diagnosis and differentiation symptomatic superior labral pathology from normal anatomy [10]. The difficulty is compounded by the degenerative changes that occur in the labrum with advanced age [4, 11].

The diagnosis of isolated SLAP lesions has historically been difficult. This has been attributed to several reasons such as the high incidence of other associated pathology. Studies of SLAP lesions suggest that most patients have pain, mechanical symptoms, notably, loss of range of motion, or inability to perform at their previous activity level [5, 6]. The poor sensitivity and specificity of clinical examination tests and difficulties with the interpretation of advanced imagery [2, 12–14] make the clinical diagnosis difficult.

When occurring in throwing athletes, SLAP lesions present an additional layer of complexity when evaluating the throwing shoulder. Through repetitive stress, elite throwers develop osseous and ligamentous adaptive changes, allowing them to reach extremes of external rotation [15].

Many surgeons including the senior author (WBS) believe that too many overhead athletes are undergoing arthroscopic SLAP repairs and that many athletes can be managed nonoperatively [16]. The operative treatment of SLAP tears remains controversial [17, 18]. SLAP repair in overhead athletes has yielded poor results and does not return the majority of athletes to their previous level of play [17, 19–22].

We must ask ourselves why the poor results and high failure rates in overhead athletes with Type II SLAP repairs Is it the failure to establish the diagnosis these athletes preoperatively and not treat them with an adequate nonoperative regimen before considering surgery? Or at the time of surgery, is it the inability of the operating surgeon to differentiate normal anatomic variants from SLAP lesions? Or is it the surgical technique that violates the rotator cuff or the improper placement of suture anchors that restricts range of motion postoperatively and disrupts overhead throwing mechanics [16]? These are all factors that will be explored in this chapter on the SLAP lesions in overhead athletes. We will discuss the anatomy and biomechanics of the glenoid labrum and its role in stability of the glenohumeral joint. This will be followed by the clinical evaluation, diagnosis, nonoperative and operative treatment of SLAP lesions in overhead athletes with tips on the surgical techniques of repairing SLAP lesions.

2. Anatomy and biomechanics

The shoulder is a mobile ball-and-socket joint with both static and dynamic stabilizers, including the glenoid with its concave surface, labrum, capsule, and its ligamentous thickenings, negative intra-articular pressure, and adhesion-cohesion of synovial fluid [23]. The glenoid labrum is fibrocartilaginous tissue with the superior labrum primarily triangular in cross section, allowing for deeper seating of the humeral head relative to the glenoid socket [24]. There is variability in this anatomy, and Higgins and Warren [25] reviewed approximately 70 peer-reviewed articles on superior labral lesions and concluded that significant anatomic variability of this region exists.

The normal superior labrum plays an essential role in providing concavity compression and thus maintaining biomechanical stability as demonstrated by the anteroinferior labrum [26]. The glenoid labrum represents the fibrocartilaginous rim between the joint capsule and the glenoid. It functions to increase the depth of articulation and, hence, the stability of the glenohumeral joint [27]. By effectively increasing the surface area available for articulation, the labrum decreases the impact stresses in the joint, especially posteriorly and inferiorly [28].

This superior labrum and biceps anchor are mobile structures during shoulder elevation, abduction, and rotation [17]. The medial rolling of the biceps anchor during abduction/external rotation (i.e., a throwing movement) may be lost after a rigid superior labrum repair resulting in shoulder pain. The long head of the biceps tendon has been suggested to have a role as a head depressor [29] or as a static stabilizer of the glenohumeral joint [30, 31]. Sakurai et al. [32] suggested that the long head of the biceps can act as a humeral head stabilizer in superior and anterior directions.

Alpantaki et al. have shown that the tendon of the long head of the biceps is innervated by a dense network of sensory sympathetic fibers, particularly in this proximal portion of the tendon, which may play a role in the pathogenesis of shoulder pain [33]. This nerve density may explain the residual pain after arthroscopic SLAP repair.

Biomechanical studies have shown that the long head of the biceps tendon acts to depress the humeral head, limit shoulder rotation, and confer anterior stability of the glenohumeral joint [34].

Other biomechanical studies have shown that destabilizing the biceps anchor leads to increased translation of the glenohumeral joint [34, 35]. When a tear of the superior labrum occurs, it is likely that symptoms are related to this increase in translation, mechanical catching of the unstable labrum within the shoulder joint, and increased forces placed on the destabilized areas during athletic activities. Previous studies have shown that SLAP lesions increase translation of the glenohumeral joint [36–38] and that those abnormal mechanics can be restored by labral repair [39]. When the labral bicipital complex is disrupted, the shoulder is allowed to go into extreme external rotation, putting increased stress on the inferior glenohumeral ligament and eventually leads to subtle instability and continued pain [40, 41].

The overhead throw motion is an extremely skillful and complex movement that is very stressful on the shoulder joint complex. The overhead throwing athletes place extraordinary demands on this complex. Excessively high stresses are applied to the shoulder joint because of the tremendous forces generated by throwers. The thrower's shoulder must be lax enough to allow excessive external rotation, but stable enough to prevent symptomatic humeral head subluxation, thus maintaining a delicate balance between mobility and functional stability. Wilk and Andrews referred to this as the "thrower's paradox," and this balance is frequently impaired, which leads to injury [42].

There are tremendous forces placed on the shoulder joint during the throwing motion. In vitro research has shown that the superior labrum must be able to withstand 262 N of shear force in the position of abduction and external rotation [43]. The arm internally rotates during the arm-acceleration phase, and the biceps force is produced to both resist shoulder distraction and elbow extension [44]. The biceps-labrum complex must be able to withstand 508 N of tensile force [43]. Fleisig et al. [45] first suggested that the tensile force produced by the biceps tendon at the ball release can lead to a SLAP tear. The forces of elite throwers approach the fatigue strength of the soft tissues of the shoulder [46]. At ball velocities of 90 MPH, the angular velocity of the shoulder approaches 7000 deg./s and the distractive force of the shoulder 950 N [47].

Numerous types of injuries may occur to the surrounding tissues during overhead throwing [42]. These superior labral tears may occur near the time of ball release, as the biceps contract to both resist glenohumeral distraction and deceleration of elbow extension [3]. Alternatively, the bicipital-labral complex may tear because of a "peel-back" mechanism as the abducted and shoulder externally rotates during the arm-cocking phase of throwing [48]. Shepard et al. [43] measured in vitro strength of the biceps-labral complex during both the distal force and peel-back mechanisms and concluded that SLAP lesions most likely occur from the repetition of both peel-back and distal forces. Other authors have demonstrated an association between posterior-superior labral lesions and contact of the rotator cuff with the arm in a cocked position [49, 50].

Assuming that in a thrower, there is an inherent adaptive increase in external rotation, it may be undesirable to restrict external rotation with surgical repair. If pitchers are unable to reach this external rotation set point or "slot," they are unable to throw with maximal velocity [15].

SLAP repair may also affect elbow function and may compromise the ability to generate elbow flexion torque in throwers to help to decelerate the elbow extensively during pitching [51]. In a study of baseball pitchers after SLAP repair versus a control group that did not have surgery, the SLAP repair group exhibited significantly less abduction and shoulder external rotation than those in the control group [51].

There is controversy as to the proper surgical technique and anchor placement for repair of type II SLAP lesions. Several biomechanical studies of Type II SLAP lesions have investigated various techniques of suture anchor placement to determine the correct repair construct. There remains no consensus on the most ideal technique for type II SLAP repairs [52]. However, looking at the biomechanical studies that have been performed and then the clinical studies, it is apparent that some anchor and suture configurations are less efficacious than others.

Bacdini et al. [53] compared single-loaded suture anchor versus double-loaded suture anchor repair and found no difference in pull-out strength. Yoo et al. determined that a mattress suture technique was inferior to a simple suture technique regarding clinical failure [54]. In contrast, the mattress suture was noted to be biomechanically superior to simple suture configurations for biceps anchor repair by Domb et al. [40]. Several studies have shown the one well-placed anchor is biomechanically sufficient [40, 53] and multiple anchors usually are not necessary. Domb et al. [40] concluded that a single anchor with a mattress suture may be the most biomechanically advantageous construct for the repair of type II SLAP lesions. The most secure knot configurations are also achieved by reversing the half-stich throws and alternating the posts [55].

Previous cadaver studies have shown an increase in external rotation with the creation of a type II SLAP tear that was correctable with a repair including anchors both anterior and posterior to the biceps anchor [39].

Cadaveric and biomechanical studies by McCulloch, Andrews, and colleagues determined that an anchor anterior to the biceps tendon had the greatest effect in decreasing external rotation [15]. The avoidance of the use of an anchor anterior to the biceps should be considered especially in baseball players and other overhead athletes where even such a small loss of external rotation would be detrimental [15]. Decrease external rotation in pitching after SLAP repair [56] is consistent with previous cadaver research that demonstrated that anchors placed anterior to the long head of the biceps tendon during SLAP repair can limit shoulder external rotation [15].

Burkart, Morgan, and colleagues suggested that in type II SLAP repairs, a suture anchor just posterior to the biceps insertion is the most important in resisting peel back forces during late cocking [57]. This is supported by a biomechanical study that shows a single anchor placed just posterior to the biceps eliminated the peel-back of the labrum [58].

The advantage of knotless versus simple repairs is still unclear. Uggen et al. [59] compared the knotless versus simple suture and found no biomechanical differences.

There is controversy and no consensus on the role of the biceps tendon in shoulder stability. One electromyographic study showed no relationship between biceps activity and active shoulder motion, suggesting that biceps muscle activity does not contribute to shoulder stability [60]. However, the absence of the long head of the biceps has been shown to result in increased shoulder instability, especially in the anterosuperior and anterior planes [30, 34]. This has been supported by Patzer et al. [30], who showed in a biomechanical study that the stabilizing effect of the superior labral complex is dependent on the attached long head of the biceps tendon. As such, there has been an emphasis on repairing lesions involving detachment of the superior labrum, especially in younger patients and high-level throwing athletes [61].

Biceps tenodesis has been proposed as an alternative or adjunct to SLAP repair [17, 62, 63]. The kinematic consequences of biceps tenodesis within the pitching motion remain largely unknown [63]. A SLAP repair preserves the glenohumeral function of the long head of the biceps tendon (LHBT), whereas biceps tenodesis removes the intra-articular portion of the LHBT and with it any function that this tendon may cause in glenohumeral kinematics [64].

3. Classification system

With the advancement of arthroscopy equipment and improved techniques, SLAP lesions have been better delineated from normal anatomy [4]. In 1990, Snyder and colleagues published their observations of superior labral tears and proposed the name SLAP lesions to indicate a more complex range of pathology related to the superior labrum extending from anterior to posterior in relation to the biceps tendon anchor [1]. The classification system proposed by Snyder et al. consisted of four subgroups of lesions categorized by the condition of the labrum and the attachment of the biceps anchor to the superior labrum and superior glenoid tubercle [65].

Type I SLAP lesions consist of fraying and fragmentation of the free edge of the superior labrum. This is often a relatively minor problem that is commonly encountered during routine arthroscopy in middle-aged and older patients [65]. Snyder considered this to be akin to a degenerative meniscus in the knee and a possible but uncommon source of clinical symptoms. In their original description, Snyder classified 21% of SLAP lesions as type I [1].

Type II lesions are by far the most common, occurring in 55% of the study patients of Snyder in their original description of SLAP lesions in 1990 [1]. In the type II SLAP lesion, the biceps anchor is significantly detached from the superior glenoid tubercle. There is usually associated fraying of the edge of the labrum, and it must be differentiated from a type I. The middle glenohumeral ligament may be considered unstable when it has a high attachment in the superior labrum and must be evaluated for security [27].

Type III SLAP lesions consist of a bucket-handle tear of a meniscoid superior labral with an otherwise normal biceps tendon attachment. This occurred in only 9% of Synder's cases in 1990 [53]. The fragment of labrum is usually mobile like a bucket handle tear of the meniscus in the knee, but it may be split in two, leaving a stub of labral tissues on either end [27]. Rarely, the middle glenohumeral ligament may be confluent with this free fragment of labrum and consequently rendered unstable [65].

Type IV SLAP lesions constituted 10% of lesions first described by Snyder in 1990 [1]. This lesion is similar to type III and includes a bucket handle tear of a meniscoid superior labrum but with the tear extending in the biceps tendon. The tendon split may be minimal or quite significant. Like the Type III lesion, the attached site of the MGHL to the labrum in the area of the tear determines the significance of the lesion regarding stability of the shoulder [65].

Snyder also described cases of combined or complex SLAP lesions. Most often, these are type III or IV lesions combined with a significantly detached biceps anchor or type II lesion. This is classified as a complex type II and III or type II and type IV lesions [65].

Moffet et al. [6] and Morgan [66] et al. and others [67] have expanded Snyder's classification scheme to include various other entities involving variations of instability patterns with congenital variations and capsular damage. Regardless of the system used, the important task of the surgeon is to carefully evaluate the superior labrum and biceps anatomy, recognize significant pathology, and be prepared to repair the SLAP lesion and associated injuries [65].

Morgan et al. [66] further subclassified type II lesions into 3 distinct subtypes—anterior, posterior, and combined anterior-posterior lesions. The clinical implications of this distinction were that superior labral tears that extend posteriorly can lead to posterior superior glenohumeral instability that overtime leads to cuff tearing [66].

The challenge with any classification system is reproducibility. Even among experienced shoulder arthroscopists, there is a lack of consensus on making a SLAP diagnosis [4]. Gobezie et al. [68] studied the inter and intra-observer reliability in the diagnosis and treatment of SLAP tears with 73 "expert surgeons." Video clips containing 22 vignettes of approximately 15 seconds duration were sent 73 shoulder surgeons and each was asked to classify the superior labral anterior posterior type using Snyder's classification system (types I–IV). The same video clips were sent again 12 months later to obtain data on intraobserver reliability. Several significant trends were noticed regarding the diagnosis and treatment responses. These included the difficulty distinguishing type III lesions from type IV lesions and the difficulty distinguishing normal shoulders from type II SLAP tears. Regarding type II SLAP tears, only 52% of surgeons made the correct diagnosis of distinguishing normal shoulders from type I and from type II SLAP lesions and making the appropriate treatment recommendations. This is a significant study and further, prospective studies need to be performed in this area and possibly better surgical education.

4. Clinical evaluation

4.1 History

The proper diagnosis of SLAP lesions can be very difficult as the clinical picture may mimic other shoulder pathology. SLAP lesions rarely occur in isolation and are often associated with other shoulder conditions such as impingement, rotator cuff tendinitis, instability, and rotator cuff tears. When occurring in throwing athletes, SLAP lesions present an additional layer of complexity when evaluating the throwing shoulder. Studies of SLAP lesions suggest that most patients have pain, mechanical symptoms, notably, loss of range of motion, or inability to perform at their previous activity level [5, 6]. The diagnosis of isolated SLAP lesions has historically been difficult, and this has been attributed to several reasons including the high incidence of other associated pathology especially in an athlete's shoulder.

It is important first to determine whether there was an acute episode of trauma or a history of repetitive use as in overhead athletes. Many others have described a fall on an outstretched arm [1, 6] as a common mechanism of injury that can cause SLAP tears. This fall can cause impaction of the shoulder with a superiorly directed force driving the humeral head against the superior labrum and the biceps anchor [65]. If the force is severe enough, a "SLAP fracture" can occur, which appears as a divot in the superior dome of the humerus more anterior that the usual posterior lateral Hill-Sachs-type instability lesion [65].

Maffet et al. [6] suggested that the most common etiology was traction on the biceps tendon. The shearing forces on the superior biceps labral complex with the long head of the biceps acting as a decelerator of the arm during the follow through phase of throwing have also been proposed as mechanism for type II SLAP tears [57, 69]. Burkhart et al. described the contracture of the posterior-inferior glenohumeral ligament in throwers causing a shift of the glenohumeral contact point posterior and superiorly, increasing the shear forces on the posterior-superior labrum, generating the "peel-back" effect and a SLAP lesion [57].

The most common complaint of symptom of patients with a SLAP lesion is some type of mechanical catching or locking of the shoulder. This occurs when the unstable labrum is trapped between the humeral head and glenoid. In case of chronic SLAP lesions, there is history of an insidious onset of shoulder pain, especially in overhead athletes. The pain may increase in severity and limit sports performance with mechanical symptoms with forceful overhead movements as in throwing or overhead sports such as volleyball and the spiking maneuver.

The biggest difficulty is differentiating a symptomatic SLAP lesion from degenerative changes of the labrum or even normal variants. Most SLAP lesions occur in the dominant arm of male, high level, overhead athletes who are younger than 40 years old [70]. Patients older than 40 years of age often have degenerative changes of the labrum, which may or not be clinically significant or pathologic [4]. Pfahler and associates [11] described the normal aging pattern of the superior labrum with normal microscopic and macroscopic changes. Significant glenohumeral arthritis or full-thickness rotator cuff tears typically do not accompany a symptomatic type II SLAP tear but rather are just a part of the entire degenerative process of the shoulder joint.

SLAP tears can also occur in the presence of a shoulder dislocation and are found as the anterior labral tear progresses superiorly to the biceps anchor and posteriorly to create a SLAP with an associated Bankart lesion.

4.2 Physical examination

The symptoms of a SLAP lesion can mimic those of impingement syndrome, pathology of the rotator cuff or the AC joint, or other shoulder disorders. It is important to remember that no single physical examination finding is pathognomonic for SLAP tears [71]. SLAP tears rarely occur in isolation and are often associated with other shoulder pathology [1, 3, 5, 6, 72–74]. Even when seen in isolation, SLAP tears may mimic impingement (52%) or even anterior instability (39%) [71, 75]. Very few studies have examined the clinical signs and symptoms of isolated SLAP lesions. In 1997, we retrospectively examined 2375 patients who underwent shoulder arthroscopy and SLAP lesions were identified in 140 shoulders. Of these 140 SLAP lesions, only 26 had no other pathology. In 23 patients who had adequate postoperative follow-up, all patients had nonspecific shoulder pain, which increased with overhead activity and mimicked rotator cuff pathology. Nine patients (39%) had a positive apprehension test with only one (4%) positive relocation test. Of the 23 patients, over one half (52%) had a positive Neer test and 35% had a positive Hawkins test. A positive Speed's test (biceps tension test) was seen in 35% and 43% who had mechanical popping and snapping in their shoulder. It is apparent that even with isolated SLAP lesions, the clinical picture can be confused with rotator cuff symptomatology.

Many studies have evaluated the sensitivity, specificity, and positive and negative predictive values as well as inter-observer and intra-observer reliability of various clinical exams with limited success [68]. In a previous study of isolated SLAP lesions of the shoulder, we found no sensitive clinical test for their detection [71]. Snyder and colleagues also determined that no single or combination of tests could conclusively and reliably predict when and what type of lesion would be found at arthroscopy [5]. They determined that the most accurate test was Speed's biceps tension test [65]. Although this test is much more suggestive for damage to the biceps tendon proper than the labrum or anchor, it may be helpful when the anchor is unstable [65].

In 1996, Liu et al. [76] described the crank test and found it to be 91% sensitive in detecting glenoid labral tears, including SLAP lesions. In 1998, O'Brien et al. [77] described the active compression test, the so-called "O'Brien test" to clinically diagnose labral tears and pathologic conditions of the acromioclavicular joint. Of 56 patients who had a positive O'Brien test result and underwent subsequent operation, 53 (95%) were found to have a labral tear.

We conducted a prospective study in 2002 to determine whether the crank or O'Brien tests were reliable tools for detecting superior glenoid labral tears. Results of diagnostic arthroscopy were compared with those of the preoperative tests and determined that the crank test had only had 46% sensitivity and was only 56% specific and the O'Brien test had only a sensitivity of 54% and 31% specificity. We determined that the O'Brien and crank tests were not sensitive clinical indicators for detecting glenoid labral tears [2]. The poor sensitivity and specificity of these clinical examination tests and others combined with difficulties with the interpretation of advanced imagery [12–14] make the clinical diagnosis of SLAP tears extremely challenging.

Cook et al. [12] conducted a prospective study to determine the accuracy of five orthopedic clinical tests for the diagnosis of SLAP lesions. The purpose of the study was to identify the diagnostic utility of the Active Compression (O'Brien's test), the biceps load II test (Kim's test), the dynamic labral shear test (O'Driscoll's test), Speed's test, and the labral tension test when diagnosing isolated SLAP lesions. Physical exam findings were compared to the findings at the time of diagnostic arthroscopy. No tests demonstrated diagnostic utility when diagnosing any SLAP lesion, including those with concomitant diagnoses. The findings suggested that each of the five stand-alone tests and clusters of tests provide minimal to no value in the diagnosis of a SLAP lesion.

Several investigators have questioned the role of SLAP lesions in shoulder stability [78]. Some have reported that SLAP lesions occur without associated glenohumeral instability [9, 60, 72, 74] while others feel that SLAP lesions are directly related to instability. The relationship between a physical finding of laxity or instability and a superior labral lesion has not been fully elucidated [78].

At the present time, there is no sensitive clinical examination test for SLAP lesions as many other pathologic conditions are associated with SLAP lesions. A high index of suspicion is necessary to accurately diagnose and treat these injuries.

4.3 Imaging

The first step in evaluating any shoulder pain is proper X-rays of the shoulder joint. This includes an anteroposterior view of the glenohumeral joint (not the shoulder as this will not give a proper view of the joint), an axillary view, and a supraspinatus outlet view. This will help rule out bony abnormalities including glenohumeral osteoarthritis, an os acromiale, or even a rare locked posterior dislocation if there is a history of significant trauma or a seizure disorder. The supraspinatus outlet view will help determine the acromial morphology (types I–III) and the thickness of the acromion, which can be important if an arthroscopic subacromial decompression is ever performed.

An MRI or an MR arthrogram is the next imaging study in evaluating shoulder pain in overhead athletes. Although a routine MRI will show significant rotator cuff pathology and glenohumeral osteoarthritis, it is not highly sensitive for detecting subtle abnormalities of the labrum such as SLAP tears or partial rotator cuff tears. An MRA is recommended as it has shown to increase the sensitivity and specificity for detecting labral tears and also partial articular sided rotator cuff tears, which is important in evaluating the overhead athlete with shoulder pain [79]. An MRI or an MRA that shows a SLAP lesion is not an automatic indication for surgery [16]. In our prospective study of U.S. Olympic Volleyball athletes, 46% of asymptomatic elite volleyball players had MRI evidence of SLAP tears but no history of complaints of shoulder problems [80]. SLAP tears are also identified on MRI in up to 48% of pitchers who are asymptomatic [23, 81]. These studies show that pathologic MRI findings in elite overhead athletes can be present. However, they are often asymptomatic. In competitive overhead athletes such as volleyball players or baseball pitchers, an MRI or MRA evidence of a SLAP lesion may not be the cause of their shoulder pain and can initially treated with nonoperative management.

5. Nonoperative treatment

Frequently, injuries of the superior labrum can be successfully treated with a well-structured and carefully implemented nonoperative rehabilitation program. The key to successful nonoperative treatment is a thorough history, clinical examination, and accurate diagnosis [42]. Typical nonoperative treatments have centered on posterior capsular stretching while maintaining glenohumeral and periscapular strength and stability [19].

The repetitive micro-traumatic stresses placed on the athlete's shoulder joint complex during the throwing motion challenges the physiologic limits of the surrounding tissues. Athletes often exhibit numerous adaptive changes that develop from the repetitive micro-traumatic stresses during overhead throwing. Alterations in throwing mechanics, muscle fatigue, muscle weakness or imbalance, and excessive capsular laxity may lead to tissue breakdown and injury [42].

Little information is available on these patients who had a successful result after nonoperative treatment [19] for SLAP lesions. Edwards et al. [19], using validated, patient-derived outcomes, showed that successful nonoperative treatment of superior labral tears results in improved pain and functional outcomes.

An overhead athlete with significant shoulder pain in their dominant arm should first be rested for 4–6 weeks and be prescribed a short course of a non-steroidal anti-inflammatory medication. During this time, a stretching program emphasizing the posterior capsule stretching should be implemented with no resistance. At 6 weeks, a structured physical therapy program is instituted working on scapulothoracic mechanics with rotator cuff strengthening. At 3 months, a gradual return to throwing or overhead activities begins, which is closely monitored by the physical therapist or athletic trainer. If the athlete is not able to return to their previous level, surgical intervention is then recommended in the hopes of returning them to their preinjury level.

6. Operative treatment

SLAP repair technique results have varied widely in the many studies reported in the literature. This is most likely explained by the variety of techniques, which have been used to address and repair the biceps labral complex/SLAP lesion to the glenoid. This includes arthroscopic debridement, the use of arthroscopic suture anchors, staples, metal screws, absorbable sutures, and biodegradable implants [5, 10, 73, 74, 82], and also biceps tenodesis and tenotomy. The high frequency at which labral injuries involve associated pathology [83] of the shoulder makes it difficult to compare the results of studies.

6.1 Debridement

Arthroscopic debridement of SLAP lesions and in particular type II SLAP lesions was originally described by Andrews and colleagues in 1985 [3]. Altchek and colleagues also reported on the arthroscopic debridement of SLAP lesions in 1992. Interestingly, at 1 year, 72% of patients noted improvement, but by 3 years, that number had dropped significantly to only 7%. They concluded and we agree that arthroscopic labral debridement is not an effective long-term solution for symptomatic relief in the overhead athlete [84].

6.2 Arthroscopic repair

Suture anchors with both simple and mattress repair techniques have been utilized with success for Type II SLAP repair [85]. Morgan et al. [66] reported that stabilization of the detached biceps anchor in shoulders with a Type-II SLAP lesion provided satisfactory clinical results and eliminated the drive through sign [86]. A mattress repair for type II SLAP repairs creates a labral bumper compared with simple repairs while both techniques result in similar biomechanical characteristics [52].

In the surgical treatment of the elite throwing athlete's shoulder with a symptomatic Type II SLAP tears, surgeons are concerned about overtightening the shoulder resulting in a loss of the necessary external rotation [15]. For this reason, it is common practice among some surgeons who treat throwers to use suture anchors placed posterior to the insertion of the long head of the biceps and to avoid anchors placed anterior to the biceps. This practice is an attempt to restore stability without compromising external rotation [15].

6.3 Tenodesis

Biceps tenodesis has been proposed as an alternative procedure to SLAP repair for overhead athletes. However, some of the results have been disappointing, with an overall return to play rate of 35% in professional baseball players and only 17% in professional baseball pitchers [62]. Boileau et al. [17] conducted a prospective study to evaluate and compare the results of biceps tenodesis and repair of isolated type II SLAP lesions. In the biceps tenodesis group, 93% (14/15) were satisfied or very satisfied and 87% (13/15) were able to return to their previous level of sports participation. Only 20% (2/10) were able to return to sports participation after SLAP repair. They concluded that arthroscopic biceps tenodesis can be considered an effective alternative to repair of a type II SLAP lesion allowing patients to return to a pre-injury level of activity of sports participation. Reviewing this paper, it is unclear what type of sports they participated in and whether or not they were overhead athletes. Also, the technique of SLAP repair, which placed an anchor anterior to the biceps tendon, which can limit external rotation, may be one of the reasons for the poor results in the SLAP repair group.

Gottschalk et al. [87] also proposed biceps tenodesis as an alternative to repair for type II and type IV SLAP tears, especially in older athletes. There remains some doubt regarding the efficacy of repairing SLAP lesions versus a biceps tenodesis in middle-aged patients [87]. In a group of 26 patients and 29 shoulders available for follow-up with an average age of 46.7 years, 89.6% were able to return to their previous level of activity. However, the vast majority of the patients in their study group were not overhead athletes.

Ek et al. [88] retrospectively reviewed 25 patients comparing type II SLAP repair versus biceps tenodesis. The 15 patients who underwent biceps tenodesis had an average age of 47 years while the 10 patients who underwent type II SLAP repair were 31 years. Both groups showed significant improvement and there was no difference in patient satisfaction, ASES scores, or return to preinjury level of sports. Tenodesis was performed in older patients who showed degenerative or frayed labrums, whereas SLAP repairs were performed in the younger group and more active patients with healthier labrums.

6.4 Tenotomy

In general, tenotomy is reserve for older, lower demand patients. With a significantly torn and degenerative SLAP lesion in an older patient, this is a very easy and quick procedure. The risk of a "Popeye" deformity in a younger, more active patient and the resultant cramping and cosmetic deformity, which can result, makes tenotomy a poor choice in overhead athletes.

6.5 Author's preferred technique

Before surgery, it is important that a long course of conservative management with a structured physical therapy and return to overhead sports program has been tried before surgery is performed in the overhead athlete. When this fails and using the proper surgical techniques, most patients can be treated successfully and return to their previous level of play. It is important that a surgeon develop a preoperative "check list" [89] to make sure that all imaging studies are up to date and available and that all the proper equipment is also available in the operating room suite. Besides having the proper anchors for a SLAP repair, the surgeon must be ready and able to address other shoulder pathology including rotator cuff tears, which can also be present at the time of surgery. **Table 1** lists all the equipment that are needed to perform the procedure. In 2019, we described the details of our preferred surgical technique along with a surgical technique video [16], which can be helpful to learn all the many steps that we will describe.

Building the proper surgical team is critical to success. This includes a skilled anesthesiologist who is comfortable with hypotensive anesthesia to control bleeding and allow for adequate visualization at the time of arthroscopy. Visualization is key to any arthroscopic surgery and excessive bleeding can prolong the procedure. A dependable circulating nurse and a skilled assistant are also critical for the procedure. It is not necessary to have another surgeon to assist but rather a good surgical technician can be trained to be an excellent assistant to hold the arthroscope in position and handle other surgical instruments.

The lateral decubitus position is preferred as it allows easier access to the anterior and anterior inferior aspect of the shoulder with less risk of cerebral hypoperfusion. We prefer general endotracheal anesthesia to maintain a secure airway, and this also allows the anesthesiologist better control of the blood pressure. All equipment should be in front of the surgeon so that he can easily check the status of all equipment including shavers, pump, and arthroscopic fluid bags to make sure everything is working properly. We also prefer a suprascapular nerve block, which is easy to administer after the patient is asleep and before beginning the procedure. We feel it is a safer block with less risk than an interscalene block.

Portal placement is key for any arthroscopic shoulder procedure. We first establish a posterior portal two finger breadths down and two finger breadths medial from the posterolateral aspect of the acromion in the interval between the infraspinatus and teres minor muscles. A 30-degree arthroscope is inserted using a 5.5 mm x 8.5 cm "J-lock" metal cannula system (Smith and Nephew/Dyonics). The shorter type of cannula is better for shoulder procedures and easier to maneuver within the shoulder

• Lateral decubitus positioning device (Hip-Grip System or Bean Bag Device)
• Shoulder suspension device with STARR Sleeve (Arthrex)
• 4.5 mm 30-degree arthroscope
• 5.5 mm x 8.5 cm metal "J-lock" arthroscopic cannula system (Smith and Nephew/Dyonics).
• 5.75 mm x 7.0 mm arthroscopic disposable cannulas (2) (Arthrex)
• Clear crystal cannula (Arthrex)
• Clear crystal cannula with a ring at end (Arthrex)
• 2.8 mm non-absorbable suture anchor (Twin-Fix/Smith and Nephew/Dyonics; Mini-Revo/Conmed/Linvatec; Fast-Fix/Arthrex) with single-loaded high-strength suture
• Crescent-shaped suture device (Conmed/Linvatec)
• #1 PDS suture-shuttle relay (Ethicon)
• 4.0 mm full radius shaver (Smith and Nephew/Dyonics)
• 4.5 mm round burr (Smith and Nephew/Dyonics)
• Shaver system (Smith and Nephew/Dyonics)
• Arthroscopic pump (Smith and Nephew/Dyonics) with lactated ringer's solution with no epinephrine

Table 1.
Proper equipment.

joint compared to the longer cannula used for knee arthroscopy. It is important to have a 5.5 mm cannula for adequate inflow through the arthroscope, which allows for adequate joint distension compared to a smaller diameter cannula (3.5–4.5 mm).

After entering the glenohumeral joint, the glenoid should be parallel to the floor and the biceps tendon is identified. Next, an anterosuperior portal needs to be created in the rotator interval between the subscapularis and supraspinatus tendons. This portal needs to be high enough in the rotator interval to allow anchor placement in the superior glenoid. If the portal is too low, the angle for anchor placement is compromised. This can be done using an outside-in technique or inside out, depending on surgeon preference. The vast majority of the time I create this portal using an inside-out technique by driving the arthroscope up into the rotator interval, removing the arthroscope but keeping the cannula in place, and then placing a smooth switching stick or rod through the posterior cannula up into the rotator interval where it then tents the skin. A small incision is then made anteriorly over the rod, and it exits out the skin. The assistant then holds the shoulder while a metal 5.5 cannula is inserted over the rod and into the glenohumeral joint.

Using an outside in technique, a spinal needle is placed percutaneously and anteriorly in the rotator interval at approximately 45 degrees to the superior tubercle under the labrum. A small skin incision is made, and the 5.5 metal cannula with a smooth obturator is used to follow the direction of the needle into the glenohumeral joint. This anterior superior portal is then hooked up to outflow (not suction!) to tubing leading to a bucket on the floor. The outflow is controlled by a clamp that the assistant periodically opens to "clear the picture" of blood or debris. The position of this portal is critical for the success of the operation and must not damage the supraspinatus tendon, which can cause postoperative pain and weakness leading to a substandard result.

After the two portals have been established, we then perform a complete 15-point diagnostic shoulder arthroscopy of the glenohumeral joint [65]. The superior labrum is part of this diagnostic examination, and careful attention needs to be made to differentiate a meniscoid-type of labrum from a type II SLAP tear (**Figure 1**). Even among experienced shoulder surgeons, this has proven to be difficult with poor inter and intra-observer reliability with only 48% of them correctly identifying type II SLAP tears [68]. Repairing a meniscoid-type of labrum or a normal labral variant can lead to a loss of external rotation, which can limit the ability of an overhead athlete to return to peak form.

Once the type II SLAP tear is properly identified, preparation for repair begins by replacing the metal 5.5 cannula in the rotator interval with a working portal, a clear, smooth 5.75 mm x 7 cm cannula (Smooth Crystal Cannula/Arthrex). This is done using a switching stick technique to maintain portal placement and avoid damage to the surrounding musculature. This working cannula has a diaphragm, which does not allow water out and therefore keeps joint distension. A 4.0 mm full radius shaver (Smith and Nephew/Dyonics) is then inserted through the anterior-superior portal for debridement of the superior glenoid of all soft tissues extending from the biceps anchor posterior to the extent of the tear.

Decortication of the superior glenoid is then performed using 4.5 mm round burr (Smith and Nephew/Dyonics) via the anterior superior portal with care not to damage the articular surfaces of the glenoid or humeral head. The burr is carefully placed between the labrum and the superior glenoid and decortication of the superior glenoid is performed (**Figure 2**) to punctate bleeding bone (**Figure 3**) and verified with the fluid being turned off. This creates a bleeding surface of growth factors from the marrow, which can enhance healing. The surgeon should stay posterior to the biceps anchor as there is no need to decorticate anteriorly.

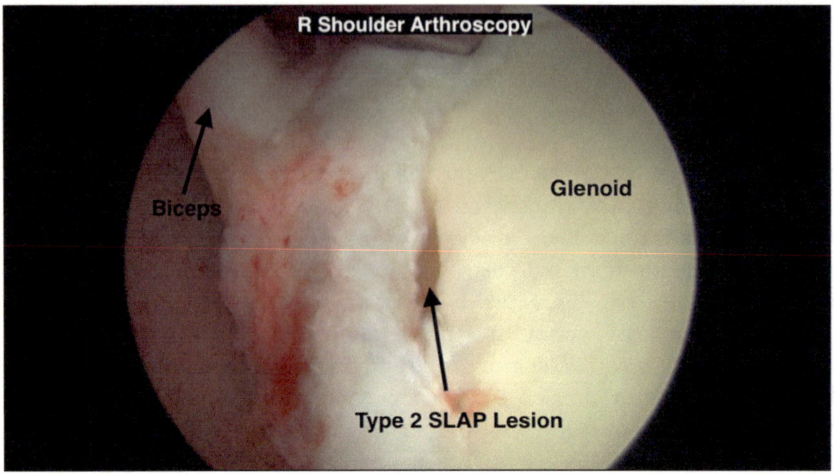

Figure 1.
A right shoulder viewing from the posterior portal in the lateral decubitus position, a type II SLAP lesion is seen here with the superior labrum along with the biceps anchor pulled away from the superior glenoid.

Once adequate decortication of the superior glenoid is performed with the burr and a bleeding bone bed has been created, a second anterior portal needs to be created for suture passage. This is created at the leading edge of the subscapularis tendon and is referred to as the mid-glenoid portal. Using an outside-in technique with a spinal needle, it is inserted at the leading edge of the subscapularis tendon high enough to allow easier passage of suture and instruments. A 5.75 mm x 7.0 mm clear cannula (Clear Crystal Cannula/Arthrex) with a ring at the end is inserted for twin anterior cannulas (**Figure 4**). This ring at the end of the cannula prevents it from "squirting" out inadvertently during the procedure.

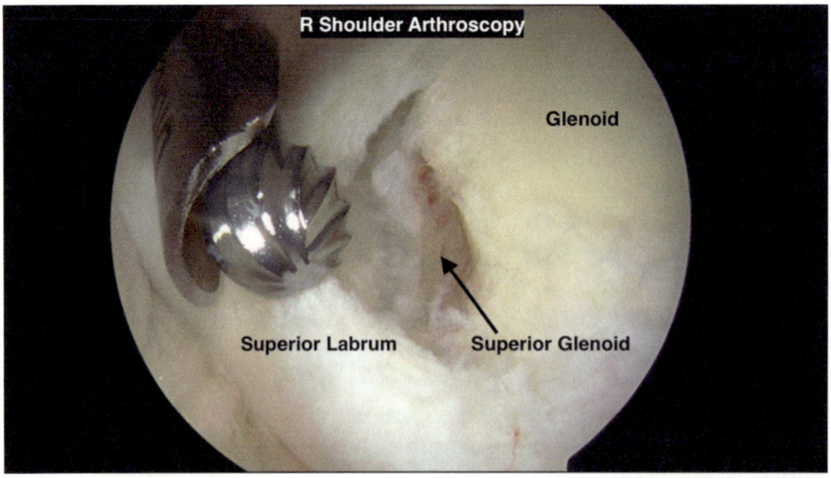

Figure 2.
A right shoulder viewing from the posterior portal in the lateral decubitus position, decortication of the superior glenoid is performed using a 4.5 mm round burr (Smith and Nephew/Dyonics) via the anterior superior portal. Care is taken not to damage the articular surfaces of the glenoid or humeral head and the burr is carefully placed between the labrum and the superior glenoid and decortication of the superior glenoid is performed.

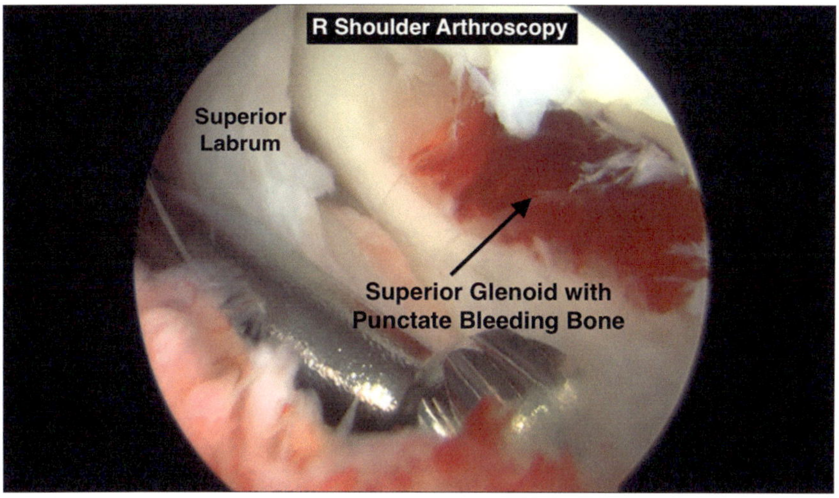

Figure 3.
A right shoulder viewing from the posterior portal in the lateral decubitus position, decortication of the superior glenoid is done until punctate bleeding bone can be seen. This is verified with the fluid being turned off and creates a bleeding surface of growth factors from the marrow, which can enhance healing. The surgeon should stay posterior to the biceps anchor as there is no need to decorticate anteriorly.

Proper anchor placement is one of the keys to success for this procedure. The anchor should be placed posterior to the biceps anchor at approximately the 12 o'clock position. There are multiple steps to anchor placement, and we recommend using them in the order described. The anterior superior portal cannula is placed just below or inferior to the biceps tendon (not above it), and 2.0 mm mini-Revo punch (Conmed/Linvatec) is inserted at a 45-degree angle into the bony bed of the area of decortication. This creates a pilot hole for the anchor. The arthroscope needs to be rotated downward to

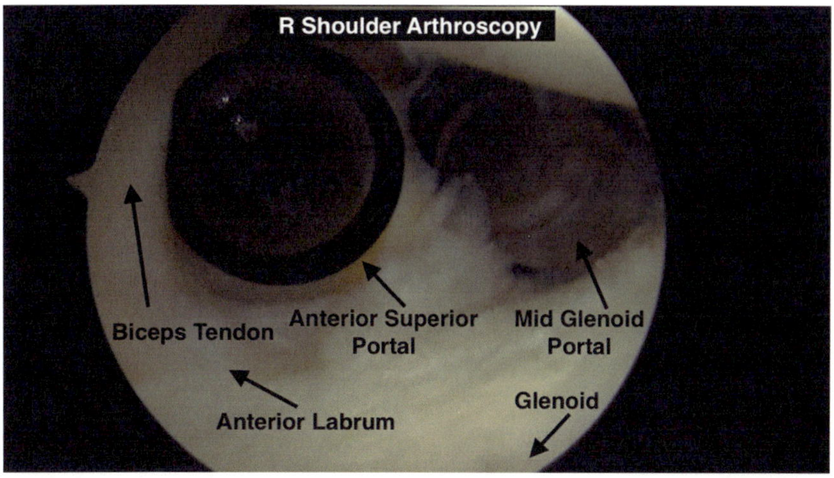

Figure 4.
A right shoulder viewing from the posterior portal in the lateral decubitus position, a second anterior portal is created for suture passage at the leading edge of the subscapularis tendon and is referred to as the mid-glenoid portal. A 5.75 mm × 7.0 mm clear cannula (Clear Crystal Cannula/Arthrex) with a ring at the end is inserted to create twin anterior cannulas. This ring at the end of the cannula prevents it from "squirting" out inadvertently during the procedure.

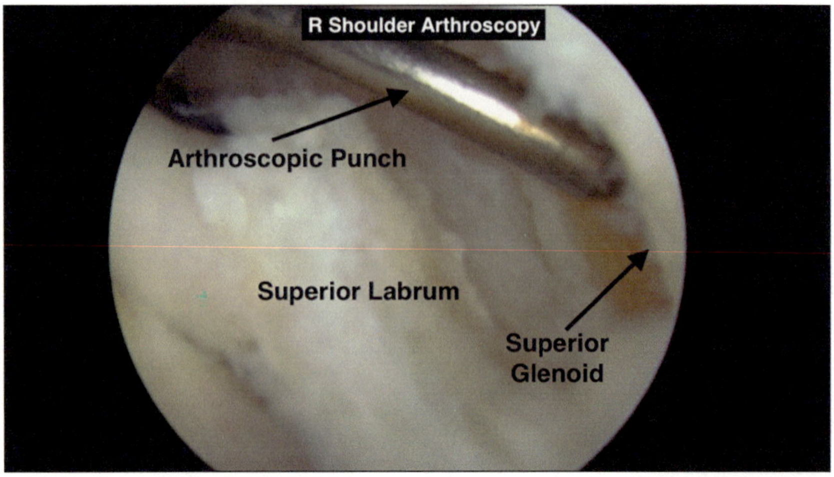

Figure 5.
A right shoulder viewing from the posterior portal in the lateral decubitus position, the arthroscope is rotated downward to the 5 o'clock position in order to adequately visualize the instruments properly. For anchor placement, a pilot hole is created at approximately the 12 o'clock position just posterior to the biceps anchor. The anterior superior portal cannula is placed just below or inferior to the biceps tendon (not above it), and a 2.0 mm mini-Revo punch (Conmed/Linvatec) is inserted at a 45-degree angle into the bony bed of the area of decortication. This creates a pilot hole for the anchor. It is important to adequately visualize the tap going into the bone and not do it blindly and skive posteriorly.

the 5 o'clock position for a right shoulder in order to adequately visualize the tap going into the bone and not skiving posteriorly (**Figure 5**) and needs to be done under direct visualization and not done blindly. Once the pilot hole has been created, the punch is removed and a 2.5 mm mini-Revo tap (Conmed/Linvatec) is inserted into the pilot hole (**Figure 6**) to create threads for the screw. We have found that in younger patients, the glenoid bone can be quite hard and self-tapping screws do not always seat properly into

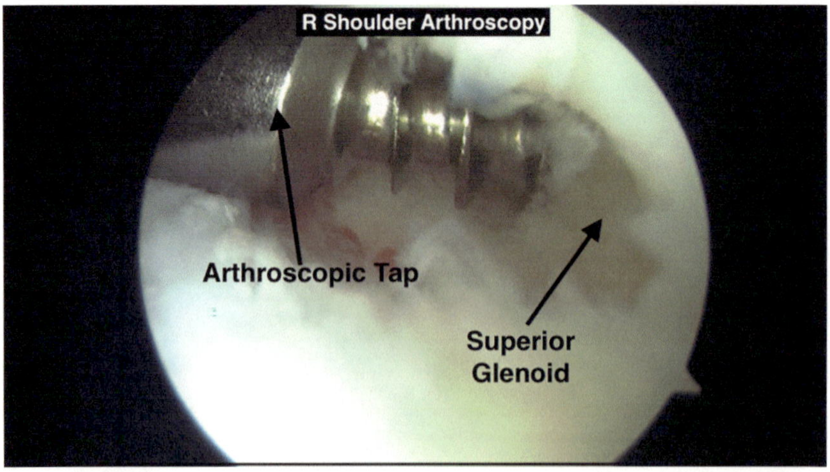

Figure 6.
A right shoulder viewing from the posterior portal in the lateral decubitus position, the pilot hole has been created and a 2.5 mm mini-Revo tap (Conmed/Linvatec) is inserted into the pilot hole to create threads for the screw. We have found that in younger patients, the glenoid bone can be quite hard and self-tapping screws do not always seat properly into the bone.

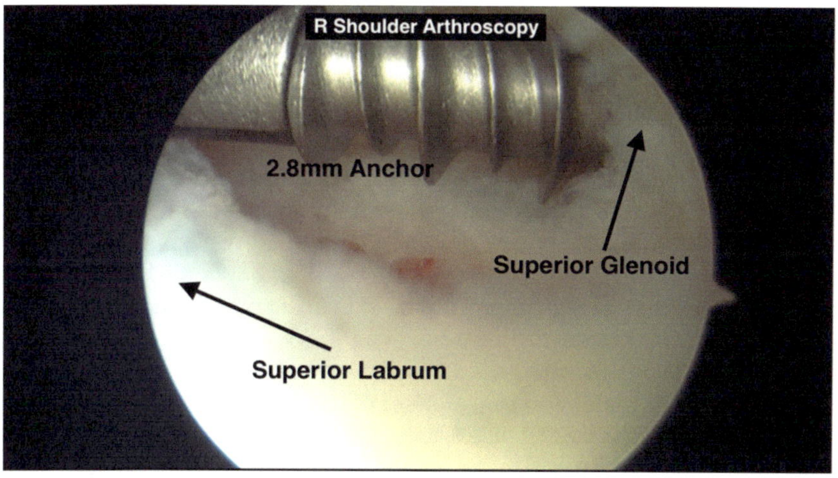

Figure 7.
A right shoulder viewing from the posterior portal in the lateral decubitus position, the tap is then removed and under direct visualization, the 2.8 mm metal anchor single loaded with a high strength suture (Twin Fix 2.8 mm/Smith and Nephew; Fast-Fix 2.8 mm/Arthrex; or Mini-Revo 2.8 mm/Linvatec/Concept) is inserted via the anterior superior portal into the superior glenoid.

the bone. A proud anchor can cause significant problems to the articular cartilage of the humeral head, so it is imperative that these anchors are well embedded into the superior glenoid. The tap is then removed and under direct visualization, the 2.8 mm metal anchor single loaded with a high strength suture (Twin Fix 2.8 mm/Smith and Nephew;

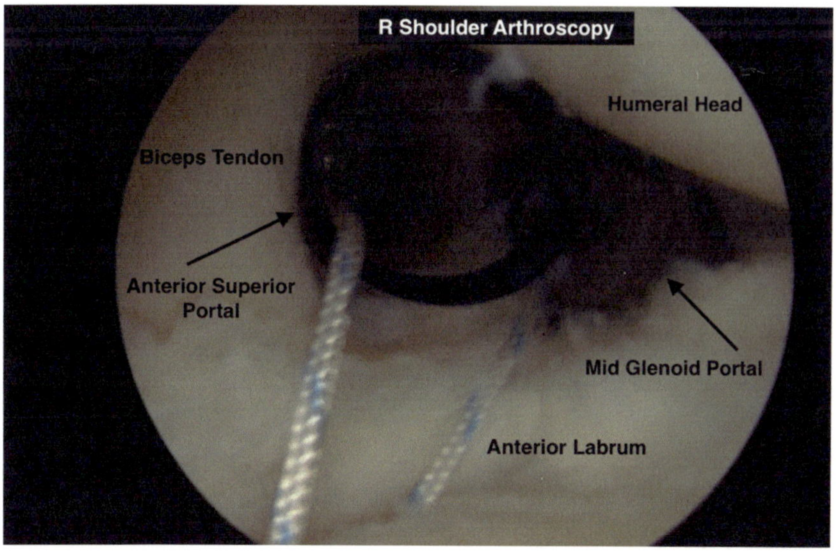

Figure 8.
A right shoulder viewing from the posterior portal in the lateral decubitus position, the arthroscope is rotated up to approximately the 1 o'clock position. A crochet hook is used for gently pulling one limb of the suture into the mid-glenoid portal. There is now one suture limb through the mid-glenoid portal and the other limb through the anterior superior portal. Suture management is also critical for a good repair. Without proper suture management, the sutures can become entangled and twisted. It is very important to keep the suture limbs separate in each portal for this part of the procedure.

Fast-Fix 2.8 mm/Arthrex; or Mini-Revo 2.8 mm/Linvatec/Concept) is inserted via the anterior superior portal into the superior glenoid (**Figure 7**). We prefer a metal anchor and have abandoned the use of bioabsorbable anchors or other plastic types of anchors because of the risk of fragmentation, synovitis, and chondrolysis.

We then test for anchor security, which is also a key step. After the anchor has been placed into the superior glenoid, the sutures are released from the driver and the driver is gently tapped out to disengage it from the anchor only a few millimeters. The sutures are then visible in the anchor and the sutures are then tugged to ensure "anchor security" and to make sure that the anchor does not come loose or become "proud." If the anchor is not secure and pulls out even a few millimeters, this can damage the articular surface of the humeral head. If by pulling on the sutures the anchor becomes loose or becomes proud, the driver can easily be slid down on top of the anchor again, re-engaged, and the anchor is seated deeper for full engagement and to make sure it will not come loose or become proud again.

Suture management is also critical for a good repair. Without proper suture management, the sutures can become entangled and twisted. After the anchor is secured into the bone, the arthroscope is rotated up from the 5 o'clock position to approximately the 1 o'clock position to view the two suture limbs coming out of the anchor. A crochet hook (not a grasper, which can damage the suture) is for gently pulling one limb of the suture into the mid-glenoid portal. There is now one suture limb through the mid-glenoid portal and the other limb through the anterior superior portal (**Figure 8**). It is very important to keep the suture limbs separate in each portal for this part of the procedure.

For suture passage and stitching, there are many devices on the market, many of them are one time use, which can be expensive. The Spectrum Soft Tissue device (Conmed/Linvatec) has different reusable attachments depending on the procedure being performed and the angle that is necessary. For a SLAP repair, we prefer the medium-sized crescent attachment, which easily fits through the 5.7 mm cannula. A #1 PDS suture (Ethicon) loaded into the back of the device, which keeps it out of the way when use the

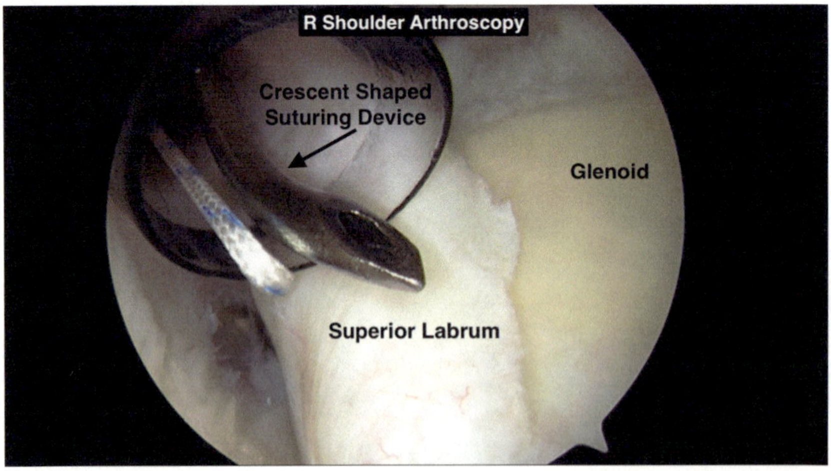

Figure 9.
A right shoulder viewing from the posterior portal in the lateral decubitus position, the Spectrum Soft Tissue device (Conmed/Linvatec) is used for a SLAP repair. We prefer the medium-sized crescent attachment, which easily fits through the 5.7 mm cannula. A #1 PDS suture (Ethicon) loaded into the back of the device, which keeps it out of the way when using the wheel to deploy the shuttle. The rotator interval portal is then placed above or superior to the biceps tendon and the Spectrum device is placed through this portal and just above the labrum. The arthroscope is rotated down into the 4 o'clock position in order to better visualize the superior labrum.

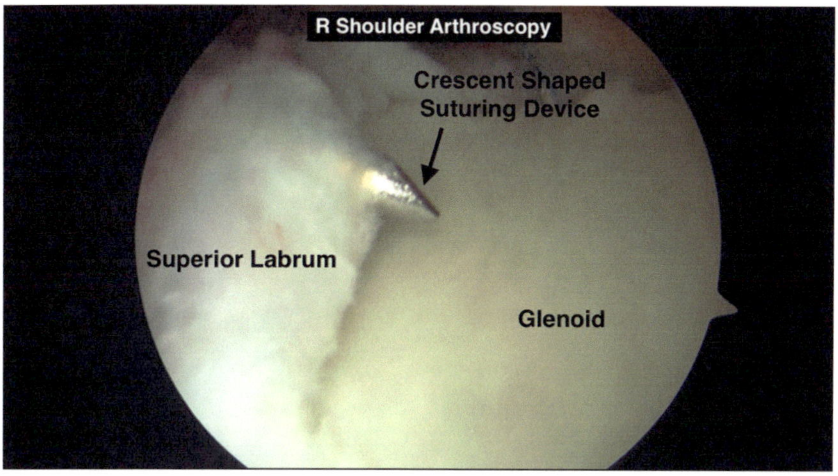

Figure 10.
A right shoulder viewing from the posterior portal in the lateral decubitus position, with careful attention not to damage the articular surface of the glenoid, the tip of the device pierces the superior labrum just posterior to the biceps tendon.

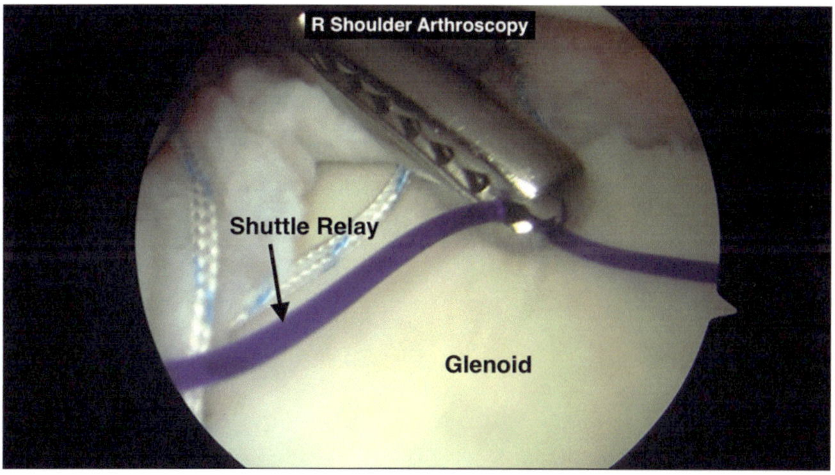

Figure 11.
A right shoulder viewing from the posterior portal in the lateral decubitus position, after the tip pierces the superior labrum the shuttle is deployed. The suture grasper via the mid-glenoid portal grasps the shuttle and pulls it out the mid-glenoid portal. A shuttling technique is used to then shuttle the mid-glenoid suture through the labrum.

wheel to deploy the shuttle. The rotator interval portal is then placed above or superior to the biceps tendon and the Spectrum device is placed through this portal and just above the labrum. The arthroscope is rotated down into the 4 o'clock position in order to better visualize the superior labrum (**Figure 9**). With careful attention not to damage the articular surface of the glenoid, the tip of the device pierces the superior labrum just posterior to the biceps tendon and the shuttle is deployed (**Figure 10**). The suture grasper via the mid-glenoid portal grasps the shuttle and pulls it out the mid-glenoid portal (**Figure 11**).

The shuttle is pulled out into the mid-glenoid portal and then clamped with a Kelly clamp to keep it from inadvertently being pulled out. The shuttle relay or PDS

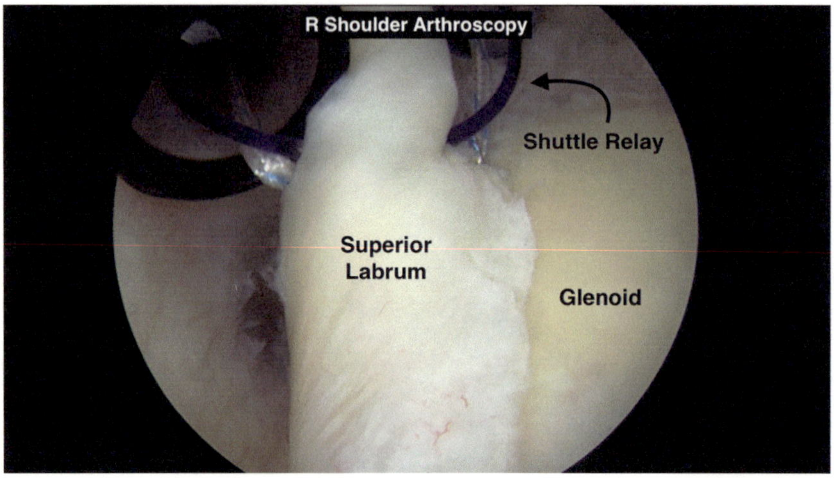

Figure 12.
A right shoulder viewing from the posterior portal in the lateral decubitus position, the PDS shuttle with the suture attached is pulled from the anterior superior portal and the suture is shuttled from the mid-glenoid portal, through the labrum, and then out the anterior superior portal.

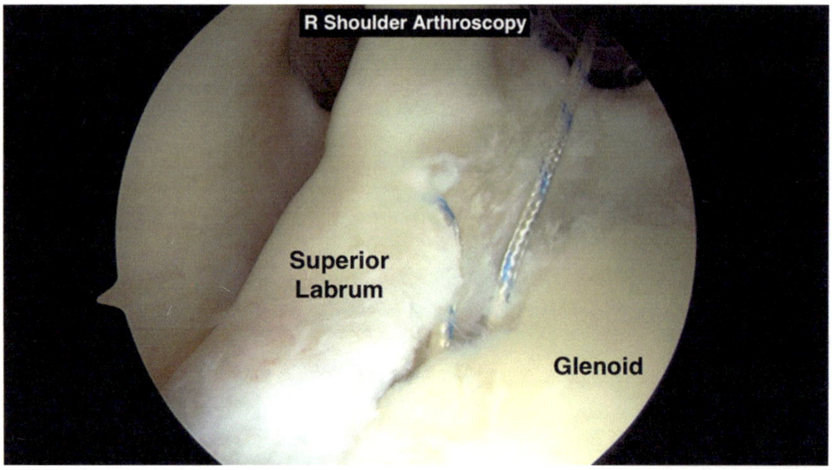

Figure 13.
A right shoulder viewing from the posterior portal in the lateral decubitus position, the first suture has been shuttled through the superior glenoid and this creates a simple knot with one limb through the labrum.

suture is then used to shuttle the first limb of the suture from the mid-glenoid portal, through the labrum, and out through the anterior superior portal. This is done by creating a "dilator knot" first on the PDS and then proximal to that creating a second knot and passing the limb of the suture through it, securing it, and then pulling on the PDS limb that is in the anterior superior portal to shuttle the first limb of the suture through the labrum (**Figures 12** and **13**). This creates a simple knot, but we prefer to repeat the process to create a mattress stitch.

Using the crochet hook placed into the mid-glenoid portal, the second limb of the suture that has not been passed through the labrum and is in the anterior-superior portal is grasped and brought into the mid-glenoid portal. The PDS suture is used again

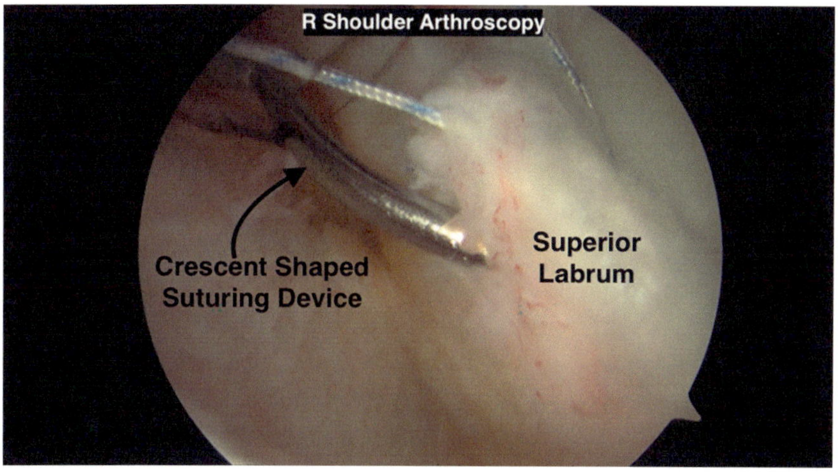

Figure 14.
A right shoulder viewing from the posterior portal in the lateral decubitus position, the arthroscope is rotated down to the 4 to 5 o'clock position and the Spectrum device with the crescent attachment is again placed into the anterior-superior portal just above the labrum. The tip of the device pierces the labrum approximately one centimeter posterior to the other limb of the suture, which has already been shuttled through the labrum.

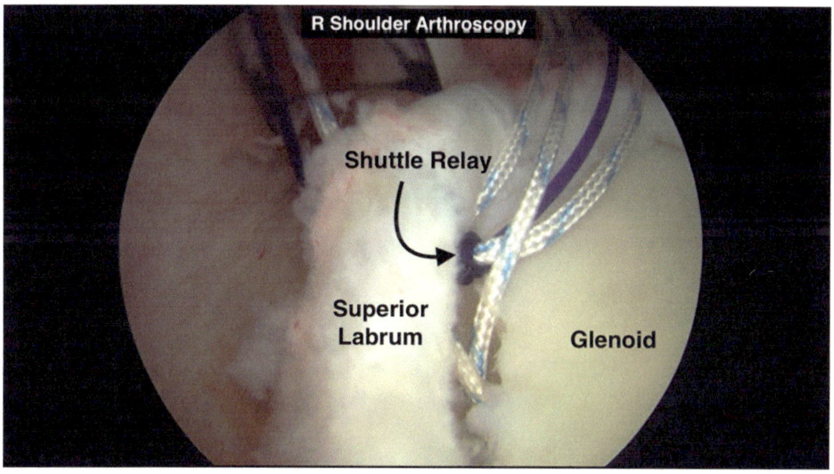

Figure 15.
A right shoulder viewing from the posterior portal in the lateral decubitus position, the process is then repeated with grabbing the shuttle from the mid-glenoid portal, bringing it out the cannula, securing the second limb of the suture outside the mid-glenoid portal with the PDS suture and shuttling the second limb through the labrum and out the antero-superior portal.

and loaded into the Spectrum device. It is important to cut away the previous knots on the PDS as these knots will prevent the PDS from sliding through the Spectrum device. The Spectrum with the crescent attachment is again placed into the anterior-superior portal just above the labrum. The tip of the device pierces the labrum approximately 1 centimeter posterior to the other limb of the suture, which has already been shuttled through the labrum (**Figure 14**). The process is then repeated with grabbing the shuttle from the mid-glenoid portal (**Figure 15**), bringing it out the cannula, securing the second limb of the suture outside the mid-glenoid portal, and shuttling the second

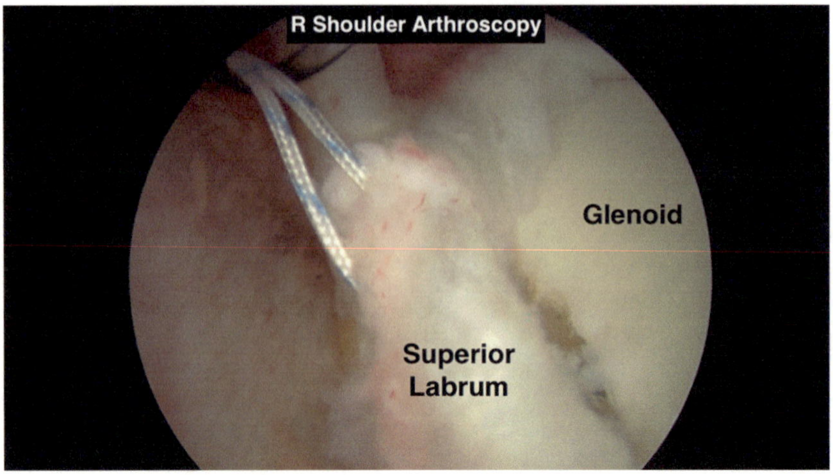

Figure 16.
A right shoulder viewing from the posterior portal in the lateral decubitus position, a mattress stitch has been created. This keeps the suture away from the articular surface and has been shown to be biomechanically stronger than a simple stitch [52, 56].

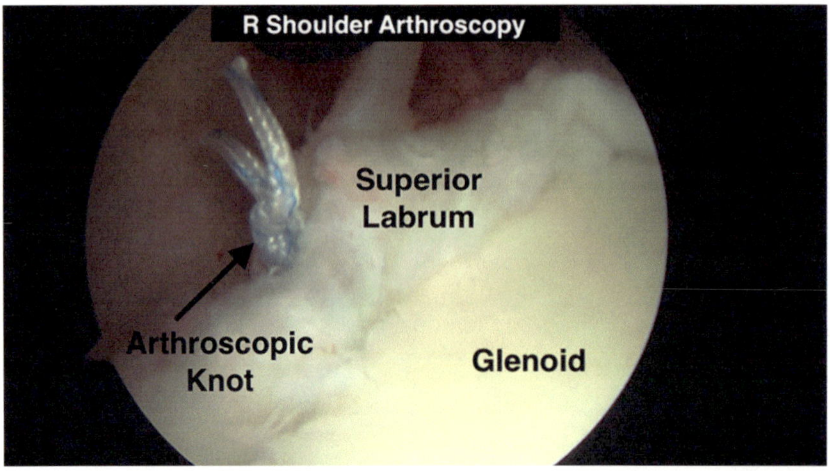

Figure 17.
A right shoulder viewing from the posterior portal in the lateral decubitus position, the knot is posterior to the biceps and the arthroscopic knot cutter cuts the suture after five half-hitches have been placed leaving a small tail at the end. With the mattress configuration, the knots are tied behind the labrum, off the articular surface, where it will not contact the humeral head or pinch between the glenoid and the humeral head.

limb through the labrum and out the antero-superior portal creating a mattress stitch (**Figure 16**). The mattress stitch keeps the knot off the articular surface and has been shown to be biomechanically stronger than a simple stitch [52, 56].

Knot tying is the final key step to a good repair. With the mattress configuration, the knots are tied behind the labrum, off the articular surface, where it will not contact the humeral head or pinch between the glenoid and the humeral head. A sliding knot is not used as sliding knots can damage and tear the labrum, which can be thin

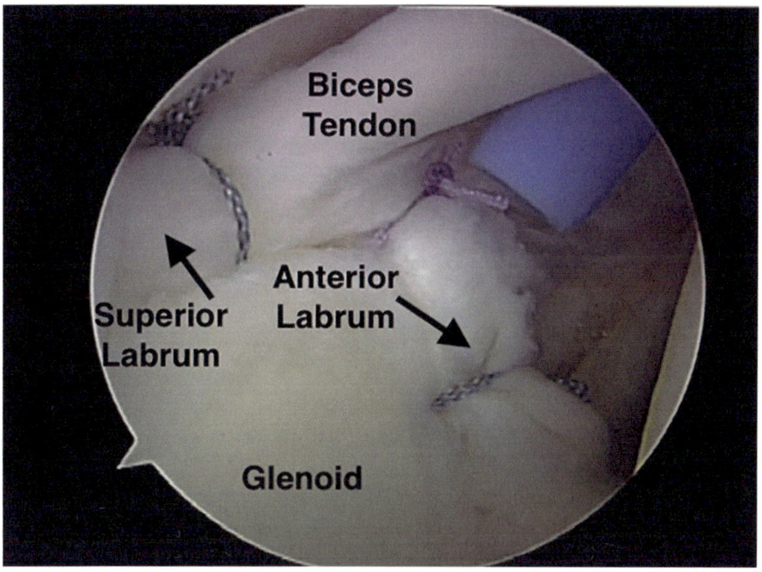

Figure 18.
A right shoulder viewing from the posterior portal in the lateral decubitus position, a different type of SLAP is depicted with anchors and sutures both posterior and anterior to the biceps anchor. Placing anchors and knots anterior to the biceps may limit external rotation by capturing the superior glenohumeral ligament which can be detrimental to the overhead athlete.

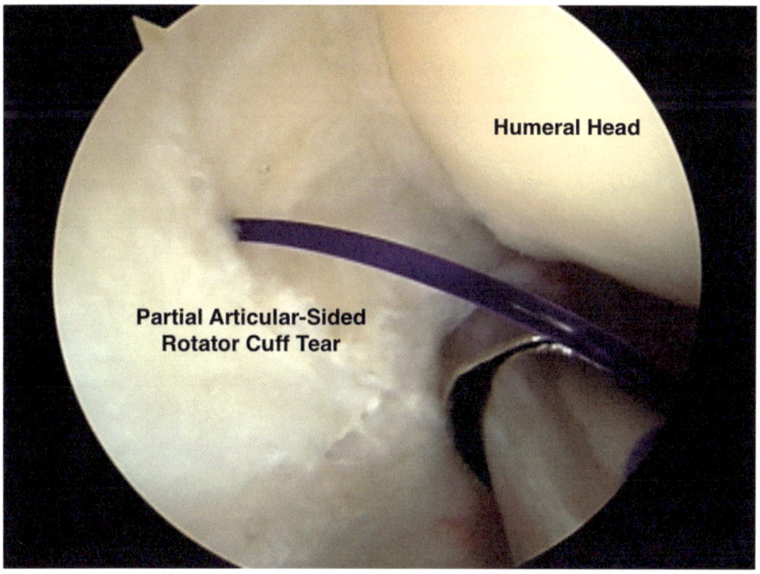

Figure 19.
A right shoulder viewing from the posterior portal in the lateral decubitus position, the arthroscope is rotated upward to about the 10 – 11 o'clock position to view the articular side of the supraspinatus tendon. If a partial articular sided cuff tear is identified in the glenohumeral joint, a marker suture technique [65] using a spinal needle can be used to place an absorbable PDS suture into the partial articular sided rotator cuff tear. This helps localize the area of the tear in the subacromial space.

in some patients. Also, sliding the knots through the anchor can damage the suture and weaken its strength. We recommend a "Revo Knot" [65] popularized by Snyder, which is a series of half-hitches. The arthroscopic knot pusher is placed via the anterosuperior portal, which is above the biceps tendon. It takes two hands to create a good arthroscopic knot so the trained assistant must be able to hold the camera in a steady position or "freeze the frame" to enable the surgeon to use two hands to create a stable knot. The knot is posterior to the biceps and the arthroscopic knot cutter cuts the suture after five half-hitches have been placed leaving a small tail at the end (**Figure 17**).

This mattress knot configuration of placing the knot behind the biceps tendon, off the articular surface, will help resist the peel back mechanism in the late phase of throwing (late cocking) [57]. Only one anchor placed posterior to the biceps is necessary [58]. Placing anchors and knots anterior to the biceps may limit external rotation by capturing the superior glenohumeral ligament (**Figure 18**), which can be detrimental to the overhead athlete.

Once the SLAP repair has been performed, it is important to address other issues inside the glenohumeral joint and the subacromial space including partial rotator cuff tears. If a partial articular sided cuff tear is identified in the glenohumeral joint, a marker suture technique [65] using a spinal needle can be used to place an absorbable PDS suture into the partial articular sided rotator cuff tear (**Figure 19**). The arthroscope is then positioned into the subacromial space. The arm holding suspension device in changed from abduction to adduction to easily facilitate entry into the subacromial space by bringing the humeral head away from the acromion. Once in the subacromial space, it is very important to evaluate for an impingement lesion and any amount of subacromial bursitis. In overhead athletes over the age of 30, it is not uncommon for them to have a significant amount of subacromial bursitis, and we recommend performing an arthroscopic subacromial decompression or "smoothing" in these athletes. We then recommend evaluating the bursal side of the rotator cuff. If a marker suture had been placed, finding the marker

• Anterior superior portal placement in the rotator interval high enough to place an anchor in the superior glenoid
• Second anterior portal at the leading edge of the subscapularis tendon created using an outside-in technique
• Decortication of the superior glenoid surface with a 4.0 mm burr to create a bleeding surface with "punctate" bleeding bone
• Never violate the supraspinatus tendon with a cannula as this can lead to residual pain and weakness in the postoperative period
• Never place an anchor anterior to the biceps tendon as this can capture the superior glenohumeral ligament and middle glenohumeral ligament leading to loss of external rotation and also tethering of the biceps tendon
• A single anchor centered at approximately the 12 o'clock position of the glenoid with a single high-strength suture is almost always adequate enough for repair
• A "Portal of Wilmington" is rarely necessary for anchor placement. If this portal is used, a cannula should not be used as this can substantially damage the rotator cuff tendon
• Always use a mattress stitch with the knot tied behind the labrum
• Always use a half-hitch knot and not a sliding knot as a sliding knot can damage the labrum

Table 2.
Key points for arthroscopic repair.

suture on the top or bursal side of the rotator cuff will help evaluate this side of the rotator cuff. If there is any significant damage to the bursal side of the rotator cuff, the surgeon has different options including debridement, a PASTA repair [65], or completing the tear and converting to a full thickness tear and repairing it. The details of this procedure are being the scope of this chapter, but shoulder surgeons who treat overhead athletes must be experienced in all of these techniques as no one technique is used all the time.

The key points for this procedure are outlined in **Table 2**.

7. Postoperative rehabilitation

Postoperatively, the SLAP repair needs to be protected for a minimum of 4 weeks before any resistive biceps is allowed. A sling is used postoperatively for only 2 weeks, but patients are asked to come out of the sling on postoperative day #1 and do elbow flexion and extension exercises along with gripping of a ball to reduce hand swelling. Pendulum exercises are started on postoperative day #2 and a formal exercise program is started 7–10 days postoperatively. Progressive resistance exercises are started at 6 weeks and a return to sports and throwing program is started at 3 months if motion is normal and patients have regained 80% of their strength. Return to sports including unrestricted overhead sports is allowed at 6 months.

8. Discussion

The published literature reveals that a significant percentage of athletes are unable to return to their prior level of athletic participation after repair of type II SLAP lesions, which is especially true for overhead athletes such a baseball players [10, 21, 22, 83, 90–92]. In baseball pitchers, the success rates for those who have undergone arthroscopic repair of Type II SLAP lesions are even poorer, ranging from 7 to 62% [10, 21, 22, 32, 83, 93–95]. Gorantla et al. [96] in a systematic review of the literature found that only 63% of overhead athletes who underwent type II SLAP repairs were able to return to sports at their previous level of competition.

Shoulder injuries in overhead athletes, especially those who throw, can be a debilitating condition that can severely limit and end the ability to participate [93]. SLAP tears can be challenging to treat in the overhead athlete. Nonoperative and operative treatments have been discussed with nonoperative treatment being the mainstay of treatment for the overhead athlete with a clinical diagnosis of a SLAP tear. As we have seen, SLAP tears can be seen in asymptomatic overhead athletes so initial nonoperative treatment will return most overhead athletes back to their pre-injury level of competition without surgery. When nonoperative treatment fails, which it can, arthroscopic surgical intervention can return most athletes to competition at or near their pre-injury level if the proper surgical techniques are used.

There have been unsuccessful outcomes with debridement alone for Type II SLAP lesions [5, 44, 84]. Arthroscopic debridement was initially recommended by some authors [3, 84], but the long-term results were disappointing. Cordasco et al. reported that arthroscopic debridement of Type II SLAP lesions was not effective with deteriorating results over 3 years. Their initial success rate was 78% at 1 year, 63% at 2 years, and only 45% at 3 years [44].

Initially, high rates of return to play were reported [97–99]. However, in these early studies of SLAP lesions, the outcome data are based largely in retrospective studies consisting of small numbers of patients using various surgical techniques and fixation options [61]. Many reports of the treatment of SLAP lesions have included patient who had other associated abnormalities making it difficult to clarify the clinical efficacy of treatment of the superior labral lesion alone [22].

Wilke, Andrews, and Meister [42] described the delicate balance of the thrower's shoulder, which has sufficient laxity to allow excessive external rotation and stability provided by the glenohumeral articulation and scapula can be easily disrupted. This has been described as the so-called "Thrower's Paradox" and disruption of this fine balance disables the throwing shoulder. The return to play (RTP) at an athlete's previous level of competition is a measure of the success of the operation.

The overhead athlete has had poor outcomes following the surgical repair of SLAP lesions reported by many different surgeons. The return to play has varied with only 63% of overhead athletes able to return to their pre-injury level [85, 96]. Other authors including Kim et al. [22] in 2002 also reported poor results of shoulder function with overhead athletes with only 22% able to return to their same level of competitiveness in their sport. Sayde et al. [85] reported that 73% of athletes were able to return to their previous level of play, but only 63% of the subset of 198 athletes who were baseball players returned to their previous level. Smith et al. [100] identified 24 major league baseball pitchers reported to have had surgery for a SLAP tear and found that 63% returned to play in the major leagues.

For baseball pitchers, the results are even worse with rates varying from 7 to 62% [10, 21, 22, 32, 83, 93–95]. Fedoriw et al. [93] reported on a case series of professional baseball players with SLAP lesions and found out that the rate of return to their previous level of play was 24% (16/68) after conservative treatment and only 23% (9/40) for those who progressed to surgery. For baseball pitchers, the results were worse and only 7% of baseball pitchers were able to return to play with surgical treatment The reasons for the high failure rates and poor results in this subgroup of overhead athletes are multifactorial and include a lack of a proper diagnosis not only preoperatively but also intra-operatively with a possible normal meniscoid variant being inadvertently repaired. Other nuances of the surgical technique could also be the explanation including anchors placed anterior to the biceps anchor, restricting external rotation, which can decrease the ability of the baseball pitcher to reach maximum torque in their pitching delivery.

Biomechanists and pitching coaches often observe that pitchers returning from injury or from surgical repair of a SLAP lesion look like they are "holding back" [51]. Pitchers in this situation demonstrate a smaller shoulder stride, less forward trunk tilt, and/or are "pushing the ball" [51]. Pushing the ball is a colloquial expression of increased shoulder horizontal abduction and increased elbow flexion seen in pitchers after SLAP repair, most likely due to the loss of external rotation.

Using electromyogram and motion analysis, it has been shown that baseball pitchers after SLAP repair have altered biomechanics including a loss of maximal external rotation of their throwing shoulder with less horizontal abduction causing a decrease in pitching velocity [51, 62]. What is it about SLAP repair that alters the pitching biomechanics resulting in a loss of pitching velocity? More likely than not, it is the technique of placing anchors anterior to the biceps anchor, overtightening the shoulder resulting in a loss of external rotation.

An MRI/MRA finding of a SLAP is not uncommon in overhead athletes and is not an indication for immediate surgery. In our prospective study of 26 elite Olympic volleyball players with no history of any shoulder problems, MRIs of their dominant shoulders showed that 17 had evidence of partial rotator cuff tears, 6 had labral tears including 4 with SLAP tears. The dominant shoulder of overhead athletes undergoes a tremendous amount of repetitive stress and is at risk for damage. However, this damage can remain asymptomatic throughout the athlete's career and any overhead athlete with shoulder pain should also initially be treated with nonoperative management [80]. Nonoperative treatment is the mainstay in overhead athletes and surgery should only be done after a long course of conservative management ranging from 3 to 6 months.

The study of Gobezie et al. [68] of 73 "expert surgeons" who were queried with video clips had a difficult time distinguishing type I from type II SLAP lesions. Only 52% make the correct diagnosis and recommended the appropriate treatment of labral repair. The poor results in the literature of arthroscopic SLAP repair may be a failure of not only diagnosis but also repair of normal variants or SLAP tears that are mistakenly misdiagnosed as normal at the time of surgery [9].

Reviewing the literature of the results of the SLAP repairs, examining the arthroscopic techniques used by different surgeons may help explain the poor results. The techniques have evolved since the original description of SLAP tears in 1985 and we now have a better understanding of the ligamentous anatomy and biomechanics of the shoulder joint. However, many surgeons did not have the benefit of these studies when they first started treated SLAP tears. With any procedure, proper portal placement, anchor placement, and knot tying are keys to a successful surgery.

In 2002, O'Brien and colleagues [90] used a trans-rotator cuff portal for surgical repair of SLAP lesions posterior to the biceps anchor. They describe the use of a cannula but state that to minimize the degree of damage to the rotator cuff, the procedure can be performed without a cannula. However, it is unclear how many patients had a cannula placed. This portal placement with a cannula referred to as the "Port of Wilmington" can damage the musculotendinous portion of the supraspinatus tendon and may explain the poor results. Using this technique, O'Brien et al. reported that only 16 of 31 patients (44%) were able to return to their preinjury level of sports. Despite the poor results, O'Brien stated that "the trans-rotator cuff technique is an effective and safe modality to address superior labral pathology." We would disagree considering the poor results reported and do not recommend violating the rotator cuff with a large cannula for anchor placement. If it is necessary to use the "Port of Wilmington" for posterior superior anchor placement, then it should be done percutaneously without the use of a cannula and using a spinal needle for direction.

Other authors have also reported poor results using a rotator cuff penetrating or trans-rotator cuff portal. In 2006, Cohen and colleagues [83] reported on isolated SLAP lesions treated with arthroscopic fixation using a bioabsorbable tack. Only 48% were able to return to their preinjury level of athletics. In those patients in which the rotator cuff was penetrated for cannula and anchor placement, only 12 of 22 patients (55%) rated their satisfaction as good or excellent. All 10 patients who reported postoperative night pain had undergone a cuff-penetrating surgical approach.

Neri et al. [10] also described a trans-rotator cuff portal for posterior SLAP lesions and reported only a 57% return to their pre-injury level of competition. They also found that the presence of a partial articular sided rotator cuff tear significantly correlated with ability to return to sport and only 13% with a partial cuff tear were able to return to their prior level of play. We do not recommend this technique of violating the rotator cuff for anchor placement, especially with a large diameter cannula but rather prefer our technique of a single anchor placed via a cannula through the rotator interval.

As we have seen from the numerous biomechanical studies that have been performed, placing an anchor anterior to the biceps tendon (**Figure 19**) can entrap the superior glenohumeral ligament (SGHL) and the middle glenohumeral ligament

(MGHL) causing a small but significant loss of external rotation [15, 61]. The biomechanical study by Morgan and colleagues in 2008 showed no advantage of placing an anchor anterior to the biceps tendon to prevent the peel-back mechanism [101].

Tension in the ligaments after SLAP repair may resolve shoulder instability but could negatively impact and affect a pitcher's ability to attain the shoulder external rotation and longitudinal abduction necessary to throw effectively [51]. The most common complication of the symptomatic type II SLAP repair has been reported as refractory post-op stiffness in forward flexion and external rotation, reported at 8.5% [15, 51]. When Katz et al. [102] looked at a cohort of failed SLAP repairs, they found out that 75% of these patient's complained of decreased range of motion.

Other authors have also noted poor results secondary to a loss of external rotation when an anchor is placed anterior to the biceps tendon. Indeed, the majority of failed SLAP repairs complain of not only pain but loss of motion [102]. Chalmers et al. in their analysis of return to play for professional baseball pitchers detected a trend toward a decrease in maximal external rotation in pitchers after SLAP repair as compared to normal controls [62].

Another key point in the arthroscopic technique of type II SLAP repair is the type of stitch configuration used. The mattress stitch with one anchor has shown to be stronger biomechanically than the use of a simple stitch with one or even two anchors [40]. This is also helps re-create the normal superior labral anatomy [52, 56].

With a mattress configuration, the knots are away from the articular surface, are less bulky, and can cause less irritation in the thrower's shoulder, reducing the risk of postoperative pain and mechanical-like symptoms in the thrower's shoulder. Even in experienced hands, these simple knots can be bulky causing significant irritation in the overhead athlete's shoulder reducing their ability to return to their normal level of play [55]. In an analysis of 11 failed SLAP repairs by Park and colleagues [103], patients complained of persistent pain and mechanical clicking in their shoulders when they returned to throwing after surgery. At the time of repeat arthroscopy in five patients, all had the knot positioned on the glenoid and caused damage the articular surface of the humeral head. Arthroscopic removal of the stitches provided pain relief and improved their ability to return to throwing. Rhee and Ha [104] described a case report of knot-induced glenoid erosion after arthroscopic suture anchor repair of a Type II SLAP lesion. The knot can be a source of continued pain after surgery so that is why we recommend a mattress configuration.

SLAP tears rarely occur in isolation [71] and other associated shoulder pathology such as chondral lesions, Bankart lesions with instability, impingement lesions, and partial or complete rotator cuff tears, which are present, may be another reason why SLAP repairs do so poorly. It is important to take a close look at the literature in that some studies that look at only the results of isolated SLAP lesions of the shoulder also have other pathology, most commonly partial rotator cuff tears, which are a confounding variable in looking at surgical results. Brockmeier et al. [61] had 24 of their 47 study patients with partial rotator cuff tears and 24 of 47 had signs and symptoms of impingement requiring a subacromial decompression. SLAP tears rarely occur in isolation and all pathology must be addressed at the time of surgery.

In an analysis of 23 elite collegiate or professional overhead athletes, Neri et al. [10] found that the presence of a partial articular sided rotator cuff tear correlated with inability to return to pain-free preinjury levels of competition. The group of patients with concomitant partial thickness rotator cuff tears demonstrated only 13% return to prior level of play, compared with 80% return in the group without tears. Brockmeier et al. [61] noted no difference in the ability to return to sporting activities in their group of 47 patients, 23 of which had a partial rotator cuff tear treated with debridement. Coexistent partial thickness rotator cuff tears did not appear to have an effect on the outcome parameters but only 74% were able to return to their preinjury level but the majority of these patients were recreational non-overhead athletes. The presence of a rotator cuff tear, even if only a partial tear, can significantly limit the ability of an overhead athlete to return their preinjury level of competition when they have an associated SLAP tear and repair.

Because of the poor results of SLAP repairs in overhead athletes, arthroscopic biceps tenodesis has been proposed as an alternative treatment to SLAP repair in the overhead athlete [17, 63, 87, 88]. In 2018, Chalmers et al. [62] reported on 17 professional baseball players who had a biceps tenodesis for a SLAP tear. Only 35% were able to return to their prior level of play and with baseball pitchers, the results were worse with only 17% able to return to their prior level of pitching.

Some studies have also implicated age as a risk factor for failure of repairs and ultimately worse activity upon return to play [17, 51]. Denard et al. [105] reported that increasing age (>40) may be a factor associated with poorer outcomes after repair of type II SLAP lesions, but the results were not statistically significant. Many of the patients in their study were worker's compensation cases. However, the results of those greater than 40 years old who had a repair of a type II SLAP lesion were 81%, similar to other studies. Among the overhead athletes in their study, 88% (15/17) were able to return to normal activities, but it does not state if they were overhead athletes or what sports they played. Worker's compensation cases had worse results with only 64% of patients (9/14) reporting satisfactory results and return to normal activities.

These results are in similar to the results of Alpert et al. [106], who showed no difference in clinical outcomes after type II SLAP repairs in patients older and younger than 40 years (surgical techniques/suture anchors placed posterior to the biceps anchor) using a technique similar to ours. Provencher et al. [107] found that type II SLAP repair in patients older than 36 years of age was associated with a significantly higher rate of failure. In their study they had a 37% failure rate and 28% revision rate. The relative risk for failure for patients older than 36 years was 3.45. However, the technique used is different from our recommended technique in that they used a transtendinous technique through the rotator cuff for anchor placement. They also used a simple stitch configuration (not a mattress stitch), which may have influenced results.

Schroder et al. [108] reported on patients who had isolated superior labral type SLAP II lesions with long-term follow-up and found no difference was observed between older patients (>40 years) and younger patients (<40 years) in terms of overall satisfaction and functional outcome scores. We have not found this to be true in our patients, and we do not use age as a factor for repairing type II SLAP lesions but rather the quality of the labrum and the activity of the patient.

We have described the technique of the arthroscopic repair of type II SLAP lesions, which has given excellent results in our patients for over 20 years. The procedure can be technically demanding but with attention to all details of the procedure, it can be reproduced and provide excellent results in overhead athletes. The two important points of not violating the rotator cuff with cannula placement and placing an anchor with a mattress suture behind the biceps are key components of a successful surgical repair. However, before proceeding with surgery, it is important to remember that not all overhead athletes with a clinical diagnosis of a SLAP by physical exam, MRI or both, need to have surgery and nonoperative measures should always be exhausted before surgery is performed.

Author details

William B. Stetson[1,2]*, Katie Lutz[1] and Kristen Reikersdorfer[1]

1 Stetson Lee Orthopaedics and Sports Medicine, Burbank, California, USA

2 Department of Orthopaedic Surgery, University of Southern California Keck School of Medicine, USA

*Address all correspondence to: wbstetsonmd@gmail.com

References

[1] Snyder SJ, Karzel RP, Del Pizzo W, Ferkel RD, Friedman MJ. SLAP lesions of the shoulder. Arthroscopy. 1990;**6**(4): 274-279

[2] Stetson WB, Templin K. The crank test, O'brien test, and routine magnetic resonance imaging scans in the diagnosis of labral tears. The American Journal of Sports Medicine. 2002;**30**:806-809

[3] Andrews JR, Carson WG Jr, McLeod WD. Glenoid labrum tears related to the long head of the biceps. The American Journal of Sports Medicine. 1985;**13**(5):337-341

[4] Rapley JH, Barber FA. Chapter 4: Labral (including Slap) lesions: Classification and repair techniques. Sports Medicine. 2013); Operative arthroscopy Fourth Edition, Johnson DH- Editor in Chief WOCTERS KLOWER 2003;**4**(Suppl 1):149-159

[5] Snyder SJ, Banas MP, Karzel RP. An analysis of 140 injuries to the superior glenoid labrum. Journal of Shoulder and Elbow Surgery. 1995;**4**(4):243-248

[6] Maffet MW, Gartsman GM, Moseley B. Superior labrum-biceps tendon complex lesions of the shoulder. The American Journal of Sports Medicine. 1995;**23**(1):93-98

[7] Handelberg F, Willems S, Shahabpour M, Huskin JP, Kuta J. SLAP lesions: A retrospective multicenter study. Arthroscopy. 1998;**14**(8):856-862

[8] Mileski RA, Snyder SJ. Superior labral lesions in the shoulder: Pathoanatomy and surgical management. The Journal of the American Academy of Orthopaedic Surgeons. 1998;**6**(2):121-131

[9] Musgrave DS, Rodosky MW. SLAP lesions: current concepts. American Journal of Orthopedics (Belle Mead, N.J.). 2001;**30**(1):29-38

[10] Neri BR, ElAttrache NS, Owsley KC, Mohr K, Yocum LA. Outcome of type II superior labral anterior posterior repairs in elite overhead athletes: Effect of concomitant partial-thickness rotator cuff tears. The American Journal of Sports Medicine. 2011;**39**:114-120

[11] Pfahler M, Haraida S, Schulz C, Anetzberger H, Refior HJ, Bauer GS, et al. Age-related changes of the glenoid labrum in normal shoulders. Journal of Shoulder and Elbow Surgery. 2003;**12**(1):40-52

[12] Cook C, Beaty S, Kissenberth MJ, Siffri P, Pill SG, Hawkins RJ. Diagnostic accuracy of five orthopedic clinical tests for diagnosis of superior labrum anterior posterior (SLAP) lesions. Journal of Shoulder and Elbow Surgery. 2012;**21**(1):13-22

[13] Kim TK, Queale WS, Cosgarea AJ, McFarland EG. Clinical features of the different types of SLAP lesions: An analysis of one hundred and thirty-nine cases. The Journal of Bone and Joint Surgery. American Volume. 2003;**85**(1):66-71

[14] Nam EK, Snyder SJ. The diagnosis and treatment of superior labrum, anterior and posterior (SLAP) lesions. The American Journal of Sports Medicine. 2003;**31**(5):798-810

[15] McCulloch PC, Andrews WJ, Alexander J, Brekke A, Duwani S, Noble P. The effect on external rotation of an anchor placed anterior to the biceps in type 2 SLAP repairs in a cadaveric throwing model. Arthroscopy. 2013;**29**:18-24

[16] Stetson WB, Polinsky S, Morgan SA, Strawbridge J, Carcione J. Arthroscopic repair of type II SLAP lesions in overhead athletes. Arthroscopy Techniques. 2019;**8**(7):e781-e792

[17] Boileau P, Parrot S, Chuinard C, Rousanne Y, Shia D, Bicknell R. Arthroscopic treatment of isolated type II SLAP lesions: Biceps tenodesis as an alternative to reinsertion. The American Journal of Sports Medicine. 2009;**37**(5):929-936

[18] Frank RM, Nho SJ, McGill KC, Grumet RC, Cole BJ, Verma NN, et al. Retrospective analysis of arthroscopic superior labrum anterior to posterior repair: Prognostic factors associated with failure. Advances in Orthopedics. 2013;**2013**:1-7

[19] Edwards SL, Lee JA, Bell JE, et al. Nonoperative treatment of superior labrum anterior to posterior tears. The American Journal of Sports Medicine. 2010;**38**(7):1456-1461

[20] Enad JG, Gaines RJ, White SM, Kurtz CA. Arthroscopic superior labrum anterior-posterior repair in military patients. Journal of Shoulder and Elbow Surgery. 2007;**16**(3):300-305

[21] Ide J, Maeda S, Takagi K. Sports activity after arthroscopic superior labrum repair using suture anchors in overhead athletes. The American Journal of Sports Medicine. 2005;**33**(4):507-514

[22] Kim SH, Ha KI, Kim SH, Choi HJ. Results of arthroscopic treatment of superior labral lesions. The Journal of Bone and Joint Surgery. American Volume. 2002;**84**:981-985

[23] Lee SB, Kim KJ, O'Driscoll SW, Morrey BF, An KN. Dynamic glenohumeral stability provided by the rotator cuff muscles in the mid-range and end-range of motion. A study in cadavera. The Journal of Bone and Joint Surgery. American Volume. 2000;**82**(6):849-857

[24] Keener JD, Brophy RH. Superior labral tears of the shoulder: Pathogenesis, evaluation, and treatment. The Journal of the American Academy of Orthopaedic Surgeons. 2009;**17**(10):627-637

[25] Higgins LD, Warner JJ. Superior labral lesions: Anatomy, pathology, and treatment. Clinical Orthopaedics and Related Research. 2001;**390**:73-82

[26] Lazarus MD, Sidles JA, Harryman DT 2nd. Matsen FA 3rd. Effect of a chondral-labral defect on glenoid concavity and glenohumeral stability. A cadaveric model. The Journal of Bone and Joint Surgery. American Volume. 1996;**78**(1):94-102

[27] Cooper DE, Arnoczky SP, O'Brien SJ, Warren RF, DiCarlo E, Allen AA. Anatomy, histology, and vascularity of the glenoid labrum. An anatomical study. The Journal of Bone and Joint Surgery. American Volume. 1992;**74**(1):46-52

[28] Karzel R, Number G, Tautenschlager E. Contact stresses during compression loading of the glenohumeral joint: The role of the glenoid labrum. Proceedings of the Institute of Medicine of Chicago. 1989;**42**:64-54

[29] Kumar VP, Satku K, Balasubramaniam P. The role of the long head of biceps brachii in the stabilization of the head of the humerus. Clinical Orthopaedics and Related Research. 1989;**244**:172-175

[30] Patzer T, Habermeyer P, Hurschler C, Bobrowitsch E, Wellmann M, Kircher J, et al. The influence of superior labrum anterior to posterior (SLAP) repair on

restoring baseline glenohumeral translation and increased biceps loading after simulated SLAP tear and the effectiveness of SLAP repair after long head of biceps tenotomy. Journal of Shoulder and Elbow Surgery. 2012;**21**(11):1580-1587

[31] Strauss EJ, Salata MJ, Sershon RA, Garbis N, Provencher MT, Wang VM, et al. Role of the superior labrum after biceps tenodesis in glenohumeral stability. Journal of Shoulder and Elbow Surgery. 2014;**23**(4):485-491

[32] Pagnani MJ, Speer KP, Altchek DW, Warren RF, Dines DM. Arthroscopic fixation of superior labral lesions using a biodegradable implant: A preliminary report. Arthroscopy. 1995;**11**(2):194-198

[33] Alpantaki K, McLaughlin D, Karagogeos D, Hadjipavlou A, Kontakis G. Sympathetic and sensory neural elements in the tendon of the long head of the biceps. The Journal of Bone and Joint Surgery. American Volume. 2005;**87**(7):1580-1583

[34] Rodosky MW, Harner CD, Fu FH. The role of the long head of the biceps muscle and superior glenoid labrum in anterior stability of the shoulder. The American Journal of Sports Medicine. 1994;**22**(1):121-130

[35] Pagnani MJ, Deng XH, Warren RF, Torzilli PA, Altchek DW. Effect of lesions of the superior portion of the glenoid labrum on glenohumeral translation. The Journal of Bone and Joint Surgery. American Volume. 1995;**77**(7):1003-1010

[36] Burkart A, Debski RE, Musahl V, McMahon PJ. Glenohumeral translations are only partially restored after repair of a simulated type II superior labral lesion. The American Journal of Sports Medicine. 2003;**31**(1):56-63

[37] McMahon PJ, Burkart A, Musahl V, Debski RE. Glenohumeral translations are increased after a type II superior labrum anterior-posterior lesion: A cadaveric study of severity of passive stabilizer injury. Journal of Shoulder and Elbow Surgery. 2004;**13**(1):39-44

[38] Mihata T, McGarry MH, Tibone JE, Fitzpatrick MJ, Kinoshita M, Lee TQ. Biomechanical assessment of type II superior labral anterior-posterior (SLAP) lesions associated with anterior shoulder capsular laxity as seen in throwers: A cadaveric study. The American Journal of Sports Medicine. 2008;**36**(8):1604-1610

[39] Panossian VR, Mihata T, Tibone JE, Fitzpatrick MJ, McGarry MH, Lee TQ. Biomechanical analysis of isolated type II SLAP lesions and repair. Journal of Shoulder and Elbow Surgery. 2005;**14**(5):529-534

[40] Domb BG, Ehteshami JR, Shindle MK. Biomechanical comparison of 3 suture anchor configurations for repair of type II SLAP lesions. Arthroscopy. 2007;**23**(2):135-140

[41] Itoi E, Kuechle DK, Newman SR, Morrey BF, An KN. Stabilising function of the biceps in stable and unstable shoulders. Journal of Bone and Joint Surgery. British Volume (London). 1993;**75**(4):546-550

[42] Wilk KE, Meister K, Andrews JR. Current concepts in the rehabilitation of the overhead throwing athlete. The American Journal of Sports Medicine. 2002;**30**(1):136-151

[43] Shepard MF, Dugas JR, Zeng N, Andrews JR. Differences in the ultimate strength of the biceps anchor and the generation of type II superior labral anterior posterior lesions in a cadaveric model. The American Journal of Sports Medicine. 2004;**32**(5):1197-1201

[44] Cordasco FA, Steinmann S, Flatow EL, Bigliani LU. Arthroscopic

treatment of glenoid labral tears. The American Journal of Sports Medicine. 1993;**21**(3):425-430 discussion 430-1

[45] Fleisig GS, Andrews JR, Dillman CJ, Escamilla RF. Kinetics of baseball pitching with implications about injury mechanisms. The American Journal of Sports Medicine. 1995;**23**(2):233-239

[46] Lesniak BP, Baraga MG, Jose J, Smith MK, Cunningham S, Kaplan LD. Glenohumeral findings on magnetic resonance imaging correlate with innings pitched in asymptomatic pitchers. The American Journal of Sports Medicine. 2013;**41**(9):2022-2027

[47] Dillman CJ, Fleisig GS, Andrews JR. Biomechanics of pitching with emphasis upon shoulder kinematics. The Journal of Orthopaedic and Sports Physical Therapy. 1993;**18**(2):402-408

[48] Burkhart SS, Morgan CD. The peel-back mechanism: Its role in producing and extending posterior type II SLAP lesions and its effect on SLAP repair rehabilitation. Arthroscopy. 1998;**14**(6):637-640

[49] Jobe CM. Posterior superior glenoid impingement: Expanded spectrum. Arthroscopy. 1995;**11**(5):530-536

[50] Walch G, Boileau P, Noel E, Donell ST. Impingement of the deep surface of the supraspinatus tendon on the posterosuperior glenoid rim: An arthroscopic study. Journal of Shoulder and Elbow Surgery. 1992;**1**(5):238-245

[51] Laughlin WA, Fleisig GS, Scillia AJ, Aune KT, Caine EL, Dugas JR. Deficiencies in pitching biomechanics in baseball players with a history of superior labrum anterior-posterior repair. The American Journal of Sports Medicine. 2014;**42**(12):2837-2841

[52] Bodulla MR, Adamson GJ, Gupta A, McGarry MH, Lee TQ. Restoration of labral anatomy and biomechanics after superior labral anterior-posterior repair: Comparison of mattress vs simple suture technique. The American Journal of Sports Medicine. 2012;**40**:875-881

[53] Baldini T, Snyder RL, Peacher G, Bach J, McCarty E. Strength of single-versus double-anchor repair of type II SLAP lesions: A cadaveric study. Arthroscopy. 2009;**25**(11):1257-1260

[54] Yoo JC, Ahn JH, Lee SH, Lim HC, Choi KW, Bae TS, et al. A biomechanical comparison of repair techniques in posterior type II superior labral anterior and posterior (SLAP) lesions. Journal of Shoulder and Elbow Surgery. 2008;**17**(1):144-149

[55] Loutzenheiser TD, Harryman DT 2nd, Yung SW, France MP, Sidles JA. Optimizing arthroscopic knots. Arthroscopy. 1995;**11**(2):199-206

[56] Dines JS, ElAttrache NS. Horizontal mattress suture with a knotless anchor to better recreate the normal superior labrum anatomy. Arthroscopy. 2008;**24**(12):1422-1425

[57] Burkhart SS, Morgan CD, Kibler WB. The disabled throwing shoulder: Spectrum of pathology part I: Pathoanatomy and biomechanics. Arthroscopy. 2003;**19**(4):404-420

[58] Seneviratne A, Montgomery K, Bevilacqua B, Zikria B. Quantifying the extent of a type II SLAP lesion required to cause peel-back of the glenoid labrum--a cadaveric study. Arthroscopy. 2006;**22**(11):1163.e1-1163.e6

[59] Uggen C, Wei A, Glousman RE, ElAttrache N, Tibone JE, McGarry MH, et al. Biomechanical comparison of knotless anchor repair versus simple

suture repair for type II SLAP lesions. Arthroscopy. 2009;**25**(10):1085-1092

[60] Yamaguchi K, Riew KD, Galatz LM, Syme JA, Neviaser RJ. Biceps activity during shoulder motion: An electromyographic analysis. Clinical Orthopaedics and Related Research. 1997;**336**:122-129

[61] Brockmeier SF, Voos JE, Williams RJ 3rd, Altchek DW, Cordasco FA, Allen AA. Hospital for Special Surgery Sports Medicine and Shoulder Service. Outcomes after arthroscopic repair of type-II SLAP lesions. The Journal of Bone and Joint Surgery. American Volume. 2009;**91**(7):1595-1603

[62] Chalmers P, Erickson B, Verma N, D'Angelo J, Romeo T. Incidence and return to play after biceps tenodesis in professional baseball players. Arthroscopy. 2018;**34**(3):747-751

[63] Chalmers PN, Trombley R, Cip J, el at. Postoperative restoration of upper extremity motion and neuromuscular control during the overhand pitch: Evaluation of tenodesis and repair for superior labral anterior-posterior tears. The American Journal of Sports Medicine. 2014;**42**(12):2825-2836

[64] Provencher MT, LeClere LE, Romeo AA. Subpectoral biceps tenodesis. Sports Medicine and Arthroscopy Review. 2008;**16**(3):170-176

[65] Snyder SJ. Shoulder Arthroscopy. Second ed. Philadelphia, Pennsylvania: Lippincott Williams and Wilkins; 2003

[66] Morgan CD, Burkhart SS, Palmeri M, Gillespie M. Type II SLAP lesions: Three subtypes and their relationships to superior instability and rotator cuff tears. Arthroscopy. 1998;**14**(6):553-565

[67] Powell SE, Nord KD, Ryu RKN. The diagnosis, classification, and treatment of SLAP lesions. Operative Techniques in Sports Medicine. 2004;**12**(2):99-110

[68] Gobezie R, Zurakowski D, Lavery K, Millett PJ, Cole BJ, Warner JJ. Analysis of interobserver and intraobserver variability in the diagnosis and treatment of SLAP tears using the Snyder classification. The American Journal of Sports Medicine. 2008;**36**(7):1373-1379

[69] Burkhart SS, Morgan CD, Kibler WB. The disabled throwing shoulder: Spectrum of pathology. Part II: Evaluation and treatment of SLAP lesions in throwers. Arthroscopy. 2003;**19**(5):531-539

[70] Rapley JH, Barber FA. Superior labrum anterior and posterior (SLAP) tears. In: Chapter 14. AANA Advanced Arthroscopy. The Shoulder. Philadelphia, Pennsylvania: Elsevier, Inc; 2010. pp. 177-187

[71] Stetson WB, Snyder SJ, Karzel RP. Long term clinical follow-up of isolated SLAP lesions of the shoulder. Architecture American Academy of Orthopaetic Surgery. 1997;**1**:161-164

[72] Glasgow SG, Bruce RA, Yacobucci GN, Torg JS. Arthroscopic resection of glenoid labral tears in the athlete: A report of 29 cases. Arthroscopy. 1992;**8**(1):48-54

[73] Resch H, Golser K, Thoeni H, Sperner G. Arthroscopic repair of superior glenoid labral detachment (the SLAP lesion). Journal of Shoulder and Elbow Surgery. 1993;**2**(3):147-155

[74] Yoneda M, Hirooka A, Saito S, Yamamoto T, Ochi T, Shino K. Arthroscopic stapling for detached superior glenoid labrum. Journal of Bone and Joint Surgery. British Volume (London). 1991;**73**(5):746-750

[75] Stetson WB, Snyder SJ, Karzel RP, Banas MP, Rahhal SE. Long-term clinical follow-up of isolated SLAP lesions of the shoulder. Arthroscopy. 1996;**12**(3):351-352

[76] Liu SH, Henry MH, Nuccion SL. A prospective evaluation of a new physical examination in predicting glenoid labral tears. The American Journal of Sports Medicine. 1996;**24**(6):721-725

[77] O'Brien SJ, Pagnani MJ, Fealy S, McGlynn SR, Wilson JB. The active compression test: A new and effective test for diagnosing labral tears and acromioclavicular joint abnormality. The American Journal of Sports Medicine. 1998;**26**(5):610-613

[78] Kim T, Queale W, Cosgarea A, McFarland E. Clinical features of the different types of SLAP lesions: An analysis of 139 cases. The Journal of Bone and Joint Surgery. American Volume. 2003;**85**(1):66-71

[79] Stetson WB, Phillips T, Meckel C, Deutsch A. The use of magnetic resonance arthrography to detect partial rotator cuff tears. The Journal of Bone and Joint Surgery. American Volume. 2005;**87**(suppl 2):81-88

[80] Lee CS, Goldhaber NH, Powell SE, Stetson WB. Magnetic resonance imaging findings in a asymptomatic elite overhead athletes. Arthroscopy. 2017;**33**(10):58-59

[81] Sheridan K, Kreulen C, Kim S, Mak W, Lewis K, Marder R. Accuracy of magnetic resonance imaging to diagnose superior labrum anterior-posterior tears. Knee Surgery, Sports Traumatology, Arthroscopy. 2015;**23**(9):2645-2650

[82] Field LD, Savoie FH 3rd. Arthroscopic suture repair of superior labral detachment lesions of the shoulder. The American Journal of Sports Medicine. 1993;**21**(6):783-790

[83] Cohen DB, Cleman S, Drakos MC, et al. Outcomes of isolated type II SLAP lesions treated with arthroscopic fixation using a bioabsorbable tack. Arthroscopy. 2006;**22**(2):136-142

[84] Altchek DW, Warren RF, Wickiewicz TL, Ortiz G. Arthroscopic labral debridement. A three-year follow-up study. The American Journal of Sports Medicine. 1992;**20**(6):702-706

[85] Sayde WM, Cohen SB, Ciccotti MG, Dodson CC. Return to play after type II superior labral anterior-posterior lesion repairs in athletes: A systematic review. Clinical Orthopaedics and Related Research. 2012;**470**(6):1595-1600

[86] Pagnani MJ, Warren RR. Arthroscopic shoulder stabilization. Operative Techniques in Sports Medicine. 1993;**1**:276-284

[87] Gottschalk MB, Karas SG, Ghattas TN, Burdette R. Subpectoral biceps tenodesis for the treatment of type II and IV superior labral anterior and posterior lesions. The American Journal of Sports Medicine. 2014;**42**:2128-2135

[88] Ek ETH, Shi LL, Tompson JD, Freehil MT, Warner JJP. Surgical treatment of isolated type II superior labrum anterior-posterior (SLAP) lesions: Repair versus biceps tenodesis. Journal of Shoulder and Elbow Surgery. 2014;**23**:1059-1065

[89] Gawande A. The Checklist Manifesto: How to Get Things Right. New York: Metropolitan Books; 2010

[90] O'Brien SJ, Allen AA, Coleman SH, et al. The trans-rotator cuff approach to SLAP lesions. Arthroscopy. 2002;**18**(4):372-377

[91] Rhee YG, Lee DH, Lim CT. Unstable isolated SLAP lesion: Clinical presentation and outcome of

arthroscopic fixation. Arthroscopy. 2005;**21**(9):1099-1104

[92] Voos JE, Pearle AD, Mattern CJ, Cordasco FA, Allen AA, Warren RF. Outcomes of combined arthroscopic rotator cuff and labral repair. The American Journal of Sports Medicine. 2007;**35**(7):1174-1179

[93] Fedoriw WW, Ramkumar P, McCulloch PC, Linter DM. Return to play after treatment of superior labral tears in professional baseball players. The American Journal of Sports Medicine. 2014;**42**:1155-1160

[94] Gilliam B, Douglas L, Fleisig G, Aune K, Mason K, Dugas J, et al. Return to play and outcomes in baseball players after superior labral anterior-posterior repairs. The American Journal of Sports Medicine. 2018;**46**(1):109-115

[95] Park S, Glousman RE. Outcomes of revision type II superior labral anterior posterior repairs. The American Journal of Sports Medicine. 2011;**39**(6):1290-1294

[96] Gorantla K, Gill C, Wright RW. The outcome of type II SLAP repair: A systemic review. Arthroscopy. 2010;**26**(4):537-545

[97] Cerynik DL, Ewald TJ, Sastry A, Amin NH, Liao JG, Tom JA. Outcomes of isolated glenoid labral injuries in professional baseball pitchers. Clinical Journal of Sport Medicine. 2008;**18**(3):255-258

[98] Park HB, Lin SK, Yokota A, McFarland EG. Return to play for rotator cuff injuries and superior labrum anterior posterior (SLAP) lesions. Clinics in Sports Medicine. 2004;**23**(3):321-334

[99] Ricchetti ET, Weidner Z, Lawrence JT, Sennett BJ, Huffman GR. Glenoid labral repair in Major League Baseball pitchers. International Journal of Sports Medicine. 2010;**31**(4):265-270

[100] Smith R, Lombardo DJ, Petersen-Fitts GR, Frank C, Tenbrunsel T, Curtis G, et al. Return to play and prior performance in Major League Baseball pitchers after repair of superior labral anterior-posterior tears. Orthopaedic Journal of Sports Medicine. 2016;**4**(12):2325967116675822

[101] Morgan RJ, Kuremsky MA, Peindl RD, Fleischli JE. A biomechanical comparison of two suture anchor configurations for the repair of type II SLAP lesions subjected to peel-back mechanism of failure. Arthroscopy. 2008;**24**:383-388

[102] Katz LM, Hsu S, Miller SL, et al. Poor outcomes after SLAP repair: Descriptive analysis and prognosis. Arthroscopy. 2009;**25**(8):849-855

[103] Park JG, Cho NS, Kim JY, Song JH, Hong SJ, Rhee YG. Arthroscopic knot removal for failed superior labrum anterior-posterior repair secondary to knot-induced pain. The American Journal of Sports Medicine. 2017;**45**(11):2563-2568

[104] Rhee YG, Ha JH. Knot-induced glenoid erosion after arthroscopic fixation for unstable superior labrum anterior-posterior lesion: Case report. Journal of Shoulder and Elbow Surgery. 2006;**15**(3):391-393

[105] Denard PJ, Lädermann A, Burkhart SS. Long-term outcome after arthroscopic repair of type II SLAP lesions: Results according to age and workers' compensation status. Arthroscopy. 2012;**28**(4):451-457

[106] Alpert JM, Wuerz TH, O'Donnell TF, Carroll KM, Brucker NN, Gill TJ. The Effeoct of age on the outcome

of arthroscopic repair of type II Sueperior labral anterior and Posterir lesions. The American Journal of Sports Medicine. 2010;**38**:2299-2303

[107] Provencher MT, McCormick F, Dewing C, McIntire S, Solomon D. A prospective analysis of 179 type 2 superior labrum anterior and posterior repairs: Outcomes and factors associated with success and failure. The American Journal of Sports Medicine. 2013;**41**(4):880-886

[108] Schroder CP, Skare O, Gjengedal E, Uppheim G, Reikeras O, Brox JI. Long term results after SLAP repair: A 5 year follow-up study of 107 patients with comparison of patients aged over and under 40 years. Arthroscopy. 2012;**28**:1601-1607

Chapter 5

Operative Hysteroscopy Complications

Anabela Serranito

Abstract

Operative hysteroscopy is a minimally invasive gynaecological procedure and is considered the gold standard for the treatment of intracavitary uterine pathology. Over the last decades, with the development of new surgical instruments, the popularity of this technique has increased with gynaecologists across the world. However, this minimally invasive technique can be associated with rare but serious complications that can lead to severe morbidity and, if not treated adequately in some cases, ultimately lead to mortality. Any gynaecologist using this procedure should not only train in the operative technique but should also acquire knowledge on what type of complications may arise whilst performing an operative hysteroscopy. The following chapter explores the diagnosis of complications associated with the operative hysteroscopy and management options.

Keywords: operative hysteroscopy, complications, uterine perforation, false passage, bleeding, fluid overload, local anaesthetic systemic toxicity, gas embolism, postoperative hematometra, postablation tubal sterilization syndrome

1. Introduction

The first reported hysteroscopy was performed in 1869 by Pantaleoni [1], making it one of the oldest reported endoscopic procedures. Hysteroscopy has greatly evolved since its primordial times and is now considered the gold standard procedure for the investigation of intrauterine pathology and subsequent treatment [2].

With the miniaturization of operative scopes and introduction of new surgical instruments, the outpatient operative hysteroscope is fast surpassing traditional in-patient hysteroscopy performed in an operating theatre [3]. This is due to the fact that office hysteroscopy offers several advantages, including shorter operating times, quicker postoperative recovery, not requiring hospital admission, no risks associated with general anaesthesia and its low cost when compared to inpatient hysteroscopy [4].

Complications during operative hysteroscopy are rare events. In a national multicentre survey in the Netherlands that analysed the complication rate in 13,600 hysteroscopic procedures (11,085 diagnostic and 2515 operative), it was reported that operative hysteroscopies had a significantly higher complications rate in relation to diagnostic procedures (i.e. 0,95% vs. 0.13%). Jansen et al. also found that more than half of the complications were entry related and that certain operative procedures carried a higher complication rate, which they associated with complexity of the technique used. Intrauterine adhesiolysis, for example, presented the highest complication rate (4,5%), with patients undergoing this procedure having a 12-fold higher complication rate when compared to those having a polypectomy [5]. In another large multicentre study in Germany that included 21,676 operative hysteroscopies, the overall complication rate was 0.22% [5]. In this study, the most common complication was uterine perforations (0.12%), followed by fluid overload (0.06%), bleeding (0.03%), bladder or bowel injury related to uterine perforation (0.02%) and infection (0.01%) [6].

Hysteroscopy in any setting is a safe procedure and surgical complication rates seem to be the same for office hysteroscopy and inpatient hysteroscopy [4]. As this technique moves into an office setting with more operative procedures being performed as an outpatient procedure, it is important to improve the training presently offered. It is imperative that training not only focus on technical skills, but also offers guidance on early diagnosis of complications and prompt management as some of these potential life-threatening complications were traditionally identified by the anaesthesiologist in a theatre setting. It is also important to further research on complications in operative hysteroscopy as the majority of knowledge presently available derives from case studies reporting on adverse outcomes.

Most complications associated with operative hysteroscopy arise during the surgery and need to be carefully discussed with the patient when explaining the procedure and surgical risks involved. However, some complications may only emerge after the procedure and are sometimes forgotten when obtaining an informed consent. It is important that these late complications also be included in the initial discussion with the patient as they may have important implications on future health issues.

2. Intraoperative complications

2.1 Vasovagal

Vasovagal reactions are a potential complication when performing hysteroscopies in an outpatient setting with incidence rates in published reports varying between 0,17% and 2,83% [7–9]. In a prospective observational study that included 2079 outpatient hysteroscopies, Agostini et al. reported that nulliparous and postmenopausal women had a higher risk of a vasovagal reaction, corresponding to 40% and 33,3% of cases, respectively. The risk is also higher when using larger diameter scopes required for operative hysteroscopy (2,83%).

These reactions are often associated with severe pain, which trigger a physiological response mediated by the parasympathetic nervous system, characterized by bradycardia and hypotension. Triggers during hysteroscopy usually include manipulation of the uterine cervix (e.g. dilatation and entry with hysteroscope) and uterine distention, but may also be triggered by severe anxiety associated with the procedure [10, 11]. If these are not managed in a timely manner, they can lead to vasovagal syncope, also known as *neurocardiogenic syncope.* Vasovagal syncope is usually preceded by prodromal symptoms that may include diaphoresis, nausea and pallor.

Management in a vasovagal reaction includes immediate removal of the stimulus, mainly by extraction of the scope, positioning the patient in reverse Trendelenburg and assessment of vitals, including blood pressure, pulse, respiratory rate and oxygen saturation. Most cases recover spontaneously within minutes. If bradycardia is persistent, an IV line should be sited and intravenous fluids started, oxygen given and local resuscitation team called [12]. If further deterioration occurs, consideration can be given to the administration of atropine.

2.2 Cervical trauma

Cervical lacerations occur when significant traction is used on handling surgical instruments applied to the cervix. In a study that included 797 operative hysteroscopes, Bigatti et al. report an incidence rate of 0,9% [13]. This type of trauma occurs mainly during the dilation of the cervix and is more frequent in women with cervical stenosis [14]. Risk factors for cervical stenosis include postmenopausal status, nulliparity, previous cervical trauma or cervical procedures. Incidence rates of cervical stenosis after cervical procedures vary between 10,2% after laser conisation and 4.3% after loop electrosurgical excision procedure [15].

Cevical tears may result in significant bleeding due to tissue trauma. Lateral cervical lacerations can extend up towards the uterus and include uterine arteries, producing substantial bleeding [14]. When applying a single-toothed tenaculum, these should be used with caution as they can easily tear the cervix [16]. Preference should be given to a double-toothed tenaculum or valsellum forceps that distribute the force applied to a broader area, providing a less traumatic grasp.

Pre-operative evaluation is important to recognise patients that are at a higher risk of cervical trauma, by identifying relevant antecedents that may increase the risk of cervical stenosis, as well as examination of cervix. In these patients, consideration should be given to the use of cervical ripening agents prior to the intervention. Studies have shown that misoprostol administered pre-operatively reduces the force required to dilate the cervix and intraoperative complications, such as cervical lacerations and false passages [17, 18]. Other options include the insertion of osmotic dilators 24 hours prior to procedure to aid in cervical softening and the use of smaller diameter scopes [19].

Management options include applying pressure with a swab on a stick to the affected area. If bleeding persists, Monsel's solution can be applied or diathermy used. In case of heavy bleeding or an extensive laceration, cervical suturing may be required.

2.3 False passage

The creation of a false passage is another complication associated with difficult entry into the uterine cavity and one of the factors associated with a failed hysteroscopy [20]. Women with cervical stenosis, abnormal uterine positions (i.e. acute anteflex- ion or retroversion), multiple caesarean sections, Asherman's syndrome or cervical fibroids are at a higher risk of false tracks [21].

False passages occur when the dilator or scope enters laterally into the muscle fibres of the cervix, instead of progressing into the uterine cavity through the internal cervical os. A high degree of suspicion should be held when the slight resistance of the dilator passing the internal cervical os is not present. On inserting the hysteroscope a criss-cross pattern of the cervical muscle fibres will be seen, instead of the normal anatomical landmarks that include a triangular cavity with bilateral tubal ostium. At this point, the operator should slowly remove the scope to correctly identify the true cervical canal for confirmation of the diagnosis.

Once the diagnosis is confirmed, the procedure should be suspended as false passages can be associated with excessive fluid absorption. Further uterine procedures should be differed for 2–3 months to allow for healing [22]. Recent papers have reported procedures being completed after the diagnosis of false passages, but case numbers are still small and further large-scale studies are required to demonstrate the safety of continuing the procedure once a false passage has occurred [21, 23].

Like any complication, prevention is essential and in high-risk patients extreme caution should be taken if proceeding with cervical dilation, using steady pressure when introducing dilators. Ideally, entry should be done with vaginoscopy with direct visualization and slow introduction of the scope through the cervical canal. If resistance is found on entry through the internal os, maintaining the inflow and closing of the outflow will increase intracervical pressure allowing for hydrodilatation of internal cervical os and allowing for the progression of the scope into the uterine cavity.

In the case of cervical stenosis, medical options such as osmotic dilators and use of cervical ripening agents (i.e. misoprostol, oestrogen in post-menopause) may be considered [24, 25]. Initial dilation with a pipelle® or entry with 2 mm diagnostic hysteroscope may also be considered before advancing with larger operative hysteroscopes [20]. Other options to navigate the stenosed cervix include surgical management (i.e. use of scissors, forceps, bipolar electrode or hysteroscopic morcellators) and ultrasound-guided entry [26–29].

2.4 Uterine perforation

Uterine perforation is the most frequent type of complication associated with hysteroscopy, with the reported rates varying between 0,12 and 3% [30]. A number of individual factors increase the risk of uterine perforation, including menopause, nulliparity, an extremely anteverted or retroverted uterus, history of a previous cervical procedure that can result in a stenosed cervical canal, intrauterine synechiae, use of gonadotropin-releasing hormone agonists and operator inexperience [5, 31].

Around 55% of uterine perforations occur during entry into the uterine cavity, whilst the remaining 45% are procedure-related [5, 32]. Patients with Asherman's syndrome have the highest risk for this type of complication, with an incidence rate as high as 10% [19]. Operator experience also seems to have an important role in the risk of uterine perforation, with around 33% of uterine perforations occurring during the surgeon's first procedure and a further 52% during the first five procedures [33]. Perforations are more frequent in patients undergoing repeat procedures, with one study demonstrating that patients undergoing a repeat endometrial ablation had an eightfold increased risk of uterine perforation [34].

Prevention begins even before the procedure with a comprehensive history that should include past medical and surgical history and completed with a thorough physical examination to help identify potential risk factors. It is important to question the patient on factors that may increase the risk of intra-abdominal adhesions, thus contributing to extreme positions of the uterus (e.g. history of endometriosis, pelvic inflammatory disease, history of peritonitis and previous abdominal surgeries including caesarean sections). Prior to beginning the procedure, it is important to examine the patient so as to determine the size and position of the uterus. One study demonstrated that 64,2% of surgeons routinely examined the patient before beginning the procedure, but 4,7% never examined the patient before the starting the procedure.

In case of uterine perforation, like any complication, early diagnosis and management can reduce severe morbidity, long-term sequalae and ultimately mortality.
On blind entry into the cavity, perforation should be suspected when a sudden loss of tissue resistance is felt or the instrument depth in the pelvis seems further than

expected. During the operative procedure, a sudden loss of intrauterine pressure or heavy bleeding should also raise concerns about possible uterine perforation. It can also be confirmed by direct visualization of intra-abdominal organs, such as a loop of the bowel or omentum, in the scope's visual field. The procedure should be suspended if there is suspicion of uterine perforation.

The anterior wall is the most frequent site for uterine perforation, followed by the cervical canal [14]. Anterior wall perforations can lead to bladder lesions, whilst lateral wall perforations are at risk of ureteral injury. Perforations occurring in the lateral walls are also more likely to cause vascular injury that can lead to broad ligament hematomas or significant intra-abdominal bleeding, with haemodynamic instability [16].

When uterine perforation occurs with a dilator, uterine sound or hysteroscope with a diameter below 5 mm and without significant bleeding, it can be managed expectantly [35]. In these cases, overnight admission for observation and a short course of antibiotics are usually the only required treatment. If there are any complaints of abdominal pain or shoulder tip pain, with haemodynamical instability, a prompt diagnostic laparoscopy is warranted. When damage occurs with larger instruments, electrosurgical or laser instruments, a systemic laparoscopic inspection of bladder, ureters, bowel and blood vessels is required to identify possible damage to these structures. In cases where organ lesion is suspected, it is crucial to obtain early support from general surgery, urology or vascular surgery depending on the type of injury. Delayed thermal injury to the bowel can manifest up to 2-week post-intervention. On discharge the patient should be informed that if any signs or symptoms of bowel perforation, such as fever, increasing pain, nausea, or vomiting, should arise they should present immediately to the emergency department.

2.5 Bleeding

Bleeding during hysteroscopy can result from entry-related complications, as previously described in this chapter, or can be procedure-related. The latter result from the transaction of vessels in the myometrium during the operative procedure. It is the second most common complication after entry-related complications, with rates varying between 0,16% and 0,61% in published reports [5, 36, 37]. Higher incidence rates are described for adhesiolysis (2.51%) and myomectomies that involve intramural components (3–4%) [38, 39].

It is often not problematic as the pressure required for uterine distention prevents loss from venous vessels. Spot electrocautery with rollerball or wire loop can be used to control bleeding from small vessels during the procedure [16]. Continuous-flow systems facilitate the removal of blood from the cavity allowing for prompt continuation of the procedure. On completing the operative procedure, intrauterine cavity pressure should be lowered slightly to identify any occult bleeding and allow for timely management.

Most operative hysteroscopies may be associated with a small amount of bleeding postoperatively, which usually stops promptly. Dilute vasopressin solution (0,05 U/mL) injected into the cervix has been shown to reduce significantly blood loss in patients with a high risk of bleeding during the procedure [40]. Vasopressin stimulates uterine contractions, thus reducing the blood loss during surgery, but it also has a direct vasoconstrictor effect and can result in serious cardiovascular complications, such as bradycardia, arrhythmias, pulmonary oedema and cardiac arrest [41, 42]. When using this medication, it is essential to ensure negative aspiration before injecting the vasopressin to avoid direct administration into a vessel resulting in systemic effects.

After completing the procedure if bleeding persists, a Foley catheter may be inserted and inflated to 20-30ml to tamponade the bleeding [43]. The balloon can be removed up to 24 h after insertion. In cases of persistent and heavy bleeding, uterine artery embolization should be considered and ultimately hysterectomy if all other interventions fail [16].

2.6 Fluid overload

Fluid overload, due to excess absorption of distention medium, occurs in 0.2–6.0% of operative hysteroscopies and is a potentially serious complication [44]. In 2018, ISGE/BSGE joint guideline on fluid management for hysteroscopy, defined fluid overload as a fluid deficit of more than 1000 ml with hypotonic solutions and 2500 ml when using isotonic solutions [45]. Risk factors that increase fluid intravasation include high intrauterine distension pressure, low mean arterial pressure, prolonged surgery, extensive surgical resection and large uterine cavities [39]. Elderly women with cardiovascular, renal or other medical comorbidities are also at a higher risk. In high risk patients the ISGE/BSGE guideline recommends using lower upper limits for defining fluid overload, with 750 ml for hypotonic solutions and 1500 ml for isotonic solutions.

This type of complication can occur with all types of distending medium and the associated pathophysiology is dependent on the type of medium used during the procedure. Fluid distending medium used in operative hysteroscopy can be broadly divided into high viscosity (e.g., dextran 70) and low viscosity, which include hypotonic (e.g. glycine 1.5%, dextrose 5% and sorbitol 3%) and isotonic media (e.g. normal saline, Ringer's lactate and 5% mannitol). High viscosity dextran 70 has fallen out of use due to its safety profile (i.e. risk of anaphylactic reactions) and potential to damage operative instruments due to crystallization [31]. In recent years, with the development of bipolar electrosurgical equipment and mechanical instruments, professional organizations have started recommending the use of isotonic media over hypotonic media due to a better safety profile [45, 46].

When intrauterine pressure exceeds the mean arterial pressure, there is an increased risk of intravasation of the distention media into the vascular system [32]. Fluid overload with hypotonic solutions will lead to hyponatremia with a rapid drop in osmolarity. In the brain, where water easily travels across the blood-brain barrier, the decreased osmolarity will allow For fluid to enter the cells resulting in cerebral oedema if left untreated. This mechanism increases intracranial pressure that can result in hypoxia and lead to cerebral herniation, resulting in irreversible brain damage [47, 48]. Premenopausal women are 25 times more likely to die or have permanent brain damage when developing hyponatraemic encephalopathy [49]. Other risks associated with specific hypotonic medium are hyperammonaemia with glycine that result in muscle aches, visual disturbances and encephalopathy. In case of using sorbital potential complications are associated with hyperglycaemia and haemolysis [14]. The use of isotonic media reduces the risk of dilutional hyponatraemia, but fluid overload can lead to hypervolemia with the accumulation of fluid in the extracellular space, giving rise to pulmonary oedema and congestive cardiac failure.

Signs of fluid overload can include nausea, vomiting, headache, agitation, confusion, visual disturbances, blindness, dyspnoea and chest pain [50]. If not identified and left untreated, the patient may develop seizures, pulmonary oedema, bradycardia and ultimately cardiopulmonary collapse.

Prevention is crucial to avoid fluid overload and careful fluid monitoring throughout operative procedures is essential. In recent years, the introduction of closed systems and automated fluid measurement systems have brought improvement as they allow for more accurate measurement of the fluid output when compared to manual measurements. During the procedure, the surgeon should use the lowest pressure to achieve a clear view of the uterine cavity, usually between 50 and 80 mmHg. In one study that included 250 operative hysteroscopies, there was no significant fluid absorption when the intrauterine pressure was kept below 80 mmHg [51].

Other important measures include obtaining baseline bloods with serum electrolytes prior to beginning surgery in high-risk patients or in those patients where a longer procedure is expected. Symptoms usually present when serum sodium concentration has fallen below 25 mmol L^{-1}, at which point the procedure should be suspended [52]. The use of intracervical injection of dilute vasopressin prior to cervical dilation has been shown to decrease fluid absorption [46]. Consideration can also be given to the pre-operative administration of gonadotrophin-releasing hormone, especially in older women, to help reduce the intravasation of fluid [45].

In cases where the patient develops fluid overload, strict fluid balance monitoring should be started and serum electrolytes measured. Patients with an asymptomatic hypervolaemia with or without hyponatraemia are easily managed with fluid restriction with or without diuretics. In patients who develop symptoms, admission to a high dependency unit may be required and early management by a multidisciplinary team (i.e. anaesthetists and intensivists). Patients should be carefully monitored for any further development of cardiac, pulmonary or cerebral changes. Management includes correction of hyponatremia with 3% hypertonic sodium chloride [45].

2.7 Neuropathies

Postoperative neuropathy is a rare complication in operative hysteroscopy as most procedures have a short duration. Nevertheless, the hysteroscopic surgeon should be aware of these and how proper patient positioning plays a crucial role in preventing this type of lesion. The most common neuropathies are related to injuries to the femoral, common peroneal and sciatic nerves [53].

The femoral nerve can be injured due to extreme angulation and compression against the inguinal ligament, caused by excessive hip flexion or extreme abduction and external rotation of the thigh when positioning the patient [54]. This type of neuropathy will result in difficulty in hip flexion/adduction and knee extension. These patients will present with inability climbing stairs in severe cases with motor damage. Patients may also complain of paraesthesia over the anterior and medial aspects of the thigh or medial aspect of the calf and foot [55].

Injury to the common peroneal nerve can occur by compression, as this nerve is in close proximity with the fibular head. Correct positioning of the patient lower limbs in padded boot stirrups can help prevent this type of lesion by avoiding direct contact of the knee or lower leg with a hard surface that can lead to nerve compression [56]. Lesions to this nerve result in the inability to perform foot dorsiflexion, lateral rotation of the ankle and extension of the toes. These lesions result in paraesthesia in the calf and dorsum of the respective foot, accompanied by foot drop.

Sciatic nerve injury, similar to the femoral nerve lesion, can occur due to excessive stretching of the respective nerve when the patient is inappropriately positioned in lithotomy with excessive hip flexion with knee extension or hip abduction with excessive external rotation of the thighs at the hips [57]. This type of neuropathy can result in paraesthesia over the posterior part of the thigh, calf and sole of the foot and cause weakness in hip extension and knee flexion [58].

2.8 Local anaesthetic systemic toxicity

Complications associated with anaesthesia in an operating theatre go beyond the scope of this chapter, but as operative hysteroscopy becomes more frequent in an outpatient setting the gynaecologist should be aware of complications arising from the use of local anaesthetics. Local anaesthetic systemic toxicity (LAST) although rare is a life-threating adverse event. Important risk factors in the hysteroscopic patient include the type and dose of local anaesthetic administered, age > 60 years, and renal and cardiac disease [59, 60].

Clinical manifestations are highly variable, but are associated with neurological and cardiac toxicity. Neurological manifestations are the most common feature, occurring usually in 68–77% of cases, and usually precede the cardiac manifestations [61]. Initial symptoms may include metallic taste, tinnitus, perioral paraesthesia, agitation and dysarthria [60]. Central nervous system toxicity can progress to seizures and ultimately coma if not managed. Cardiac signs usually manifest initially as excitation (i.e. hypertension, tachycardia or ventricular arrhythmias), and posteriorly as depression (i.e. bradycardia, conduction block and asystole) [62].

Toxicity with local anaesthetic can occur with the unintentional intravascular injection or administration of toxic doses. An important preventative measure is to aspirate before injecting the local anaesthetic to confirm that it is not being directly administrated into a blood vessel. The use of premixed syringes with epinephrine also helps reduce systemic absorption. Gynaecologists should be aware of the maximum doses for the different types of local anaesthetic [63].

If any symptoms of LAST should develop prompt consideration should be given to initiating general resuscitation measures. Administration of the local anaesthetic should be immediately stopped stop and further assistance requested. Intravenous access should be sited, standard monitoring with cardiac monitoring started, the emergency trolley should be made available and local anaesthetic/resuscitation team contacted. In severe cases, treatment with 20% intravenous lipid emulsion may be required [61].

2.9 Gas embolism

Gas embolism during operative hysteroscope is a rare complication, but extremely fatal with a mortality rate of up to 46% [64]. The pathological mechanism associated with a gas embolism is complex and triggered by the entry of gas into the systemic venous system when a pressure gradient is created between the surgical site and the right atrium [65, 66]. In operative hysteroscopy, gas can derive directly from the room air or from gas products subsequent to electrosurgical vaporization. A lethal dose can range from 3 to 5 ml/kg. With room air lethal doses can be as low as 50 ml, due to the fact that it is rich in nitrogen that is less soluble than carbon dioxide or oxygen [53, 67].

During operative hysteroscopy, air can be inadvertently introduced into the uterus due to inappropriate purging of distention fluid systems pre-operatively, multiple entries into the womb during the surgical procedure which can inject air into the cavity or in cases where there is extensive vascular lesion during procedure or cervical trauma and air can directly enter the venous system when the cervix and vagina are left open. When positioning a patient in Trendelenburg, a pressure gradient is created, facilitating the entry of gas into the incised or open veins, as the patient's head is lower than the surgical site thus increasing venous return to heart and any air bubbles present.

During hysteroscopic procedures, the intrauterine pressure created by distention fluid can reach a pressure of up to 100 mm-hg, which surpasses the mean venous pressure. This creates a dangerous gradient that facilitates fluid absorption directly from the cavity, but also the entry of any air bubbles present in the cavity into the venous system. Dyrbye et al. demonstrated that during operative hysteroscopy gas embolism was not dependent on the type of electrosurgical equipment used, but the grade of the gas embolism was more severe when the intravasation of the distension fluid surpassed one litre [68].

When entering the venous system, the gas bubbles travel to the right ventricle and can progress further to the pulmonary circulation. In the right ventricle, larger volumes of gas can occlude the outflow tract and pulmonary artery, leading to cardiovascular collapse. Likewise, when smaller amounts of gas bubbles travel to the pulmonary circulation, it can lead to pulmonary vasoconstriction, increased pulmonary artery pressure, increased resistance to right ventricular outflow, and subsequently right ventricle failure [69]. There is also a reduced ventricular preload, with a subsequent decrease in left cardiac output that leads to systemic cardiovascular failure [70]. Gas emboli can also trigger an intense inflammatory response that results in bronchoconstriction and pulmonary capillary leakage leading to pulmonary oedema and alveolar collapse [68].

During an office hysteroscopy, the gynaecologist should consider an air embolism in the differential diagnosis when the patient complains of a sudden onset of chest pain or difficulty breathing, as this can be the presenting symptom in 20–52% [63]. On pulmonary auscultation, wheezing or rales can be detected, as signs of bronchospasm and pulmonary oedema. The classic sign in cases of air embolism is the 'mill wheel' murmur, due to intracardiac air emboli [71]. A decrease in oxygen saturation can be identified in 30–72% of patients. In patients under general anaesthetic, gas embolism presents with a fall in the end-tidal CO_2, decrease in saturation of peripheral oxygen and cardiovascular symptoms [64].

In case of any suggestive symptoms or signs, the gynaecologist should have a high degree of suspicion as early identification and prompt management is crucial for patient survival. The procedure should be halted immediately to avoid further entry of air into the venous circulation. The surgeon ought to remove all instruments, and deflate the uterus and occlude the cervical os (e.g. uterine dilator and wet swabs) to avoid further entry of gas. It is also important to place the patient in reverse Trendelenburg to reduce the passage of further air emboli to the heart. The patient should additionally be placed in the left lateral position (Durant's Manoeuvre), in an attempt to move the gas emboli into the right atrium away from the right ventricular outflow tract [72]. At this point, it is crucial to initiate basic life support and that the emergency rapid response team be contacted promptly.

Prevention is a crucial step in avoiding this serious complication. During operative hysteroscopy in an office setting, patients should be monitored with pulse oximetry and if there are any signs of decreased oxygen saturation, accompanied by bradycardia or tachycardia, consideration should be given to suspending the procedure immediately. Before beginning the procedure, the surgeon should ensure that the irrigation system is fully purged of all air bubbles. When dilating the cervix, leaving the last dilator in the cervix until inserting the hysteroscope will avoid the entry of room air into the cavity. During the procedure, the surgeon should not place the patient in Trendelenburg position and limit instrument exchanges to a minimum (e.g. removal and reinsertion of the resectoscope during a procedure). Whilst performing the procedure distension pressures should be kept to the minimum required for adequate vision [63]. Pre-operative priming with GnRH agonists to reduce venous sinuses and the administration of cervical vasopressin preoperatively may help reduce the degree of intravasation during the procedure, thus reducing the risk of gas embolism [22, 73].

3. Post-operative complications

3.1 Infection

Complications associated with infection after an operative hysteroscope are rare events and the incidence ranges from 0.3% to 1,6% [74]. These include urinary tract infections, endometritis, pyometra and pelvic inflammatory disease [31].

Women with a history of pelvic inflammatory disease seem to be at an increased risk of developing infectious complications. Other risk factors are associated with the duration and type of intervention. The risk is higher in patients undergoing longer procedures, in hysteroscopic interventions with extensive endometrial destruction that may leave necrotic tissue fragments in the uterine cavity and surgeries that require multiple reinsertions of the operative instruments through the cervix [16].

Studies have demonstrated that the use of prophylactic antibiotics provides no statistical difference in relation to the incidence of postoperative infections [75–77]. Antibiotic prophylaxis is required in women with cardiac conditions at risk for endocarditis and in those patients with insertion of laminaria for cervical dilatation [19]. Some authors also recommend the administration of antibiotics in women with a history of pelvic inflammatory disease [16, 19].

Management of post-hysteroscopic infections complications should include broad-spectrum antibiotics and patients usually respond within 48 h of beginning treatment.

In patients with pyrexia, leukopenia and abnormal liver function tests not responding to antibiotics, although extremely rare, disseminated herpes should be considered. Price et al. describe a fatal case of fulminant hepatic failure in a healthy woman after a hysteroscopy due to herpes simplex virus [78], demonstrating the importance of differing hysteroscopic procedures if active genital herpes is identified.

3.2 Postoperative hematometra

Postoperative hematometra is a complication that occurs mainly after endometrial ablation/resection or intrauterine adhesiolysis for Asherman's syndrome [19]. Its incidence rate is estimated to be between 1 and 3% in patients undergoing endometrial ablation [79, 80]. Postoperative hematometra can develop centrally or in the cornual areas.

The patient is usually amenorrhoeic and presents with cyclic pelvic pain during the menstrual phase of the cycle. Symptoms can begin a few weeks after the procedure, with some patients presenting up to 16 months after the intervention. Hematometra occurring centrally result from the regeneration and sloughing of residual endometrium behind a cervical or lower uterine segment stenosis resulting from the previous hysteroscopic procedure [81]. In cornual hematometra, there is usually both a proximal and distal cornual obstruction that does not allow for decompression of the menstrual bleeding and patient will complain of homolateral pelvic pain [82].

Diagnosis is made by pelvic ultrasound, whilst the patient is symptomatic, but in cases of smaller cornual hematometra pelvic MRI may be required. In most cases, central hematometra treatment is simple requiring only cervical dilatation [83]. In recurrent cases, stent placement may be considered. Treatment of cornual hematometra involves a higher degree of complexity, with a high risk of uterine perforation due to difficulty in access, extensive adhesions and also due to the fact that the myometrium in these areas is thinner. Hysteroscopic treatment should be done under ultrasound guidance and the remaining endometrium should be resected/ablated to prevent recurrence. In case of recurrence of cornual hematometra, hysterectomy should be considered.

In order to reduce the risk of postoperative hematometra some authors recommend that when performing endometrial resection or ablation the destruction of the endometrium be terminated at the lower uterine segment, avoiding trauma to the internal cervical os that can lead to cervical stenosis.

3.3 Post-ablation tubal sterilization syndrome

Post-ablation sterilization syndrome (PATSS) is another complication associated with focal-residual endometrial tissue in uterine cornea with retrograde menstruation into an occluded tube, resulting in a hemosalpinx. It was first described by Townsend et al. in 1993 and later confirmed by Webb et al. [84, 85]. The true incidence of this syndrome is unknown with the reported incidence rates ranging from 3 to 10%, but it is believed to be underestimated as it may go undiagnosed [86, 87].

Similarly, for cornual hematometra women, PATSS will present with lateral or bilateral pelvic pain coinciding with the menstrual period. On physical examination, when symptomatic, the patient may have significant adnexal tenderness, but with no significant adnexal mass. Symptoms may start as early as 2 months post-procedure, but in one study with a 10 year follow-up some patients were diagnosed with symptoms presenting as late as 20 months after the procedure [86].

A high degree of suspicion is required in symptomatic women with a history of tubal ligation, as ultrasound may be reported as normal in cases with minimal hemosalpinx. In these cases, a T2 image-weighted MRI will aid in identifying the hemosalpinx. When diagnostic exams are performed out of the menstrual cycle, findings may be reported as normal as blood in the fallopian tube may be absorbed [80]. As this is a rare and fairly unknown pathology, the radiologist should be made aware of the clinical impression when ordering diagnostic exams.

Treatment involves laparoscopic salpingectomy and hysteroscopic adhesiolysis to prevent further cornual hematometra recurring. Salpingectomy should be performed bilaterally as there are reports of contra-lateral recurrence [39]. In cases of recurring pelvic pain, consideration should be given to a hysterectomy.

When performing endometrial ablation with first-generation equipment, the destruction of endometrial tissue in the cornual area may be challenging, due to concerns of uterine perforation in these areas where the myometrial thickness is the thinnest. MRI studies performed on women who underwent endometrial ablation with rollerball demonstrated that 95% had persistent endometrial tissue, most frequently identified in fundal area close to the ostium [85]. Second generation equipment, with shorter operating times and less complications, have gained popularity over the last few years, but also seem to be associated with PATSS [88, 89].

3.4 Intrauterine adhesions

Intrauterine adhesions (IUA) or synechiae are a significant long-term complication in women undergoing operative hysteroscope, especially in those still wishing for future pregnancies. The incidence of post-operative adhesions is dependent on the type and extent of the hysteroscopic procedure performed. In a randomized prospective study, Taskin et al. found that the incidence of IUA on a second-look hysteroscopy was 3.6% after polypectomy, 6.7% in metroplasties, 31.3% after a single myo-mectomy and as high as 45.5% in patients undergoing multiple myomectomies [90].

IUA result when there is damage to the basal layer of the endometrium with opposing uterine walls coalescing together forming adhesions that can result in a partial or total obliteration of the uterine cavity [91]. Patients will frequently complain of menstrual irregularities that include amenorrhea or hypomenorrhea, but may also include dysmenorrhea due to retrograde menstruation [92]. IUA are also an important risk factor for infertility, miscarriage, premature rupture of membranes, caesarean section due to non-cephalic presentation, low birth weight and increased risk of admission to neonatal intensive care unit [93, 94].

Although historically hysterosalpingography was used for diagnosis, presently hysteroscopy is considered the gold standard as it permits not only diagnosis, with direct inspection of the cavity to evaluate the extent of the process, but also allows for treatment during the same procedure. Multiple management approaches to adhesiolysis have been published including expectant management, hydro-dissection of thin adhesions and use of mechanical instruments, such as scissors or use of electrosurgery [92]. Recurrence rates vary from 20 to 23% in simple cases, but can be as high as 48,9% to 62,5% in cases with extensive synechiae [95, 96].

Prevention of adhesion formation is the most relevant part of any operative hysteroscopy, especially in fertile women undergoing extensive intrauterine procedures. Numerous approaches have been proposed for the prevention of IUA adhesions, but the numbers of cases included in study groups are usually small and there are few comparative studies. Prevention begins before the surgery and patients should be informed of the risks of IUA prior to any operative hysteroscopy. In cases of hysteroscopy for suspected IUA, the patient should be informed about the clinical risks involved when undertaking adhesiolysis, including uterine perforation. The patients should also be warned that normal cavity anatomy may not be obtained and that multiple procedures may be required due to extensive adhesions and recurrence.

In a recent systemic review that included 4953 women who had undergone adhesiolysis, it was demonstrated that these patients had an increased risk of ectopic pregnancy, pregnancy loss, placenta previa, placenta abruption, premature rupture of membrane, placenta accreta, neonatal death and stillbirth when compared to women in the general population [97].

During adhesiolysis, some authors favour the use of mechanical instruments over electrosurgical energy due to concerns about theoretical endometrial damage caused by instruments that use energy sources [98]. Recent studies have demonstrated lower adhesion rates when using bipolar instruments, which is attributed to a selective resection process, with less endometrial damage, when compared to monopolar equipment. More research is required to compare the different techniques including the newer mechanical instruments.

Post-procedure preventative measures include early repeat second-look hysteroscopy [99], the use of mechanical barriers (i.e. intrauterine device [100], intrauterine balloon stent [101] and folley catheter [102]), use of hyaluronic acid, and other anti-adhesion barriers [103, 104] and medical therapies [105] to aid in the restoration of the endometrium. More recently the use of stem cells has been proposed to help regenerate the endometrium [106].

3.5 Pregnancy following endometrial resection and endometrial ablation

Endometrial resection or ablation has become a largely disseminated technique for treating heavy menstrual bleeding refractory to medical management, with several benefits over the more invasive hysterectomy [107, 108]. Multiple techniques have been developed, but the principle remains the same across the different methods, aiming for the complete destruction of the endometrium down to the basalis layer.

Endometrial ablation is not contraceptive and when pregnancy does occur in the remaining refractory endometrium, it can be associated with multiple adverse outcomes resulting from implantation in a scarred uterus. The number of pregnancies after endometrial ablation has been increasing and the reported rates range from 0.24% to as high as 5.2%, with the highest rate being for patients having undergone balloon ablations [109, 110]. In a recent systemic review by Kohn et al., the majority of cases occurred in patients who had undergone an endometrial ablation with a first-generation technique (83% in trials and cohorts and 71% in case studies), with smaller numbers after a second-generation technique (17% in trials and cohorts and 19% in case studies) [109].

Any pregnancy occurring after an ablative procedure should be considered a high-risk pregnancy and added surveillance is required. The risk of ectopic is high 6–7%, when compared to the 2% in the general population and may occur in rare locations such as cervical and cornual locations [111–113]. In patients who have undergone an endometrial ablation and have a positive pregnancy test, an early pregnancy scan is required to exclude an ectopic pregnancy. Pregnant women with a history of endometrial ablation are at a higher risk of miscarriage, preterm premature rupture of membranes, premature delivery, intrauterine growth restriction, caesarean section and abnormal placentation [110, 114].

One of the major concerns in pregnant patients with a history of an endometrial ablation are of a *placenta accreta spectrum disorder*. Kohn et al. found in their review that included 258 post-ablation pregnancies, an incidence rate of approximately 12%. In this same group, 81% underwent a hysterectomy and 40% were complicated by a postpartum haemorrhage. Taking this into consideration, these patients should be reviewed in tertiary centers that have experience in diagnosing placenta accreta spectrum disorders and the delivery should take place in units with surgeons that have experience in postpartum hysterectomies.

3.6 Uterine rupture

Operative hysteroscopy has greatly evolved over recent years, reducing the need for traditional open surgery for the treatment of uterine septa, synechiae and fibroids. Nevertheless, information on the long-term obstetrical outcomes after these types of procedures is limited and most published research is derived from case reports on individual cases with adverse outcomes.

Uterine rupture is an extremely rare, but devastating complication resulting in adverse outcomes for both mother and foetus. In recent decades, there have been an increasing number of reports on uterine rupture in patients who underwent an operative hysteroscopy that was complicated by a uterine perforation [115–118]. Other reported risk factors related to hysteroscopy that can result in a uterine rupture during pregnancy include metroplasty, adhesiolysis and myomectomy [119–123].

It is hypothesized that these types of procedures weaken the myometrium ultimately leading to a uterine rupture during pregnancy when the muscle fibers are required to stretch so as to accommodate the growing pregnancy [124]. In a review by Sentilhes et al., it was found that monopolar energy had been used in 9 of the 13 reported cases (69%) [125]. It was theorised that the use of electrosurgery during hysteroscopy may provoke thermal damage to tissue leading to the weakening of the muscle fibers that can eventually result in a uterine rupture [126].

When obtaining consent for operative hysteroscopy in women of reproductive age, it is important to counsel women on the obstetrics risks that may result from the procedure. There is no consensus on the safe interval between procedure and pregnancy with reported cases of a uterine rupture occurring between 1-month and 5-year post-procedure [125]. Nevertheless, women who have undergone extensive operative hysteroscopy are at a high risk of adverse obstetric outcomes, especially when there has been a uterine perforation and will require increased surveillance during their pregnancy.

Author details

Anabela Serranito
Coombe Women and Infant's University Hospital/Midlands Regional Hospital Portlaoise, Dublin, Ireland

*Address all correspondence to: adserranito@gmail.com

References

[1] Pantaleoni DC. On endoscopic examination of the cavity of the womb. Medicine Press Crinic. 1869;**8**:26

[2] Mairos J, Di Martino P. Office hysteroscopy. An operative gold standard technique and an important contribution to patient safety. Gynecological Surgery. 2016;**13**(2):111-114

[3] Campo R, Santangelo F, Gordts S, Di Cesare C, Van Kerrebroeck H, De Angelis MC, et al. Outpatient hysteroscopy. Facts, Views & Vision in ObGyn. 2018;**10**(3):115

[4] Mak JN, Imran A, Burnet S. Office hysteroscopy: Back to the future! Climacteric. 2020;**23**(4):350-354

[5] Jansen FW, Vredevoogd CB, Van Ulzen K, Hermans J, Trimbos JB, Trimbos-Kemper TC. Complications of hysteroscopy: A prospective, multicenter study. Obstetrics & Gynecology. 2000;**96**(2):266-270

[6] Aydeniz B, Gruber IV, Schauf B, Kurek R, Meyer A, Wallwiener D. A multicenter survey of complications associated with 21,676 operative hysteroscopies. European Journal of Obstetrics, Gynecology, and Reproductive Biology. 2002;**104**(2): 160-164

[7] Agostini A, Bretelle F, Ronda I, Roger V, Cravello L, Blanc B. Risk of vasovagal syndrome during outpatient hysteroscopy. The Journal of the American Association of Gynecologic Laparoscopists. 2004;**11**(2):245-247

[8] Bellingham FR. Outpatient hysteroscopy problems. The Australian & New Zealand Journal of Obstetrics & Gynaecology. 1997;**37**(2):202-205

[9] Cicinelli E, Parisi C, Galantino P, Pinto V, Barba B, Schonauer S. Reliability, Feasibility, and Safety of Minihysteroscopy with a Vaginoscopic Approach: Experience with 6,000 Cases. Fertility and sterility. 2003;**80**(1):199-202

[10] Cicinelli E, Didonna T, Ambrosi G, Schönauer LM, Fiore G, Matteo MG. Topical anaesthesia for diagnostic hysteroscopy and endometrial biopsy in postmenopausal women: A randomised placebo-controlled double-blind study. British Journal of Obstetrics and Gynaecology. 1997;**104**(3):316-319

[11] Tsai PS, Chen CP, Tsai MS. Perioperative vasovagal syncope with focus on obstetric anesthesia. Taiwanese Journal of Obstetrics & Gynecology. 2006;**45**(3):208-214

[12] Salazar CA, Isaacson KB. Office operative hysteroscopy: An update. Journal of Minimally Invasive Gynecology. 2018;**25**(2):199-208

[13] Bigatti G. The shaver technique for operative hysteroscopy. In: Hysteroscopy. Cham: Springer; 2018. pp. 635-648

[14] Nabi S. Hysteroscopic complications. European Journal of Medical and Health Sciences. 2022;**4**(3):13-16

[15] Baldauf JJ, Dreyfus M, Ritter J, Meyer P, Philippe E. Risk of cervical stenosis after large loop excision or laser conization. Obstetrics & Gynecology. 1996;**88**(6):933-938

[16] Cooper JM, Brady RM. Intraoperative and early postoperative complications of operative hysteroscopy. Obstetrics and Gynecology Clinics of North America. 2000;**27**(2):347-366

[17] Waddell G, Desindes S, Takser L, Beauchemin MC, Bessette P. Cervical

ripening using vaginal misoprostol before hysteroscopy: A double-blind randomized trial. Journal of Minimally Invasive Gynecology. 2008;**15**(6):739-744

[18] Al-Fozan H, Firwana B, Al Kadri H, Hassan S, Tulandi T. Preoperative ripening of the cervix before operative hysteroscopy. Cochrane Database of Systematic Reviews. 2015;**4**

[19] Isaacson KB. Complications of hysteroscopy. Obstetrics and Gynecology Clinics of North America. 1999;**26**(1):39-51

[20] Relph S, Lawton T, Broadbent M, Karoshi M. Failed hysteroscopy and further management strategies. The Obstetrician & Gynaecologist. 2016;**18**(1):65-68

[21] Hota T, Abuzeid OM, Raju R, Holmes J, Hebert J, Abuzeid MI. Management of false passage complication during operative hysteroscopy. Middle East Fertility Society Journal. 2022;**27**(1):1-8

[22] Glasser MH. Hysteroscopy: Managing and minimizing operative complications. OBG Management. 2005;**17**(2):42-57

[23] Song D, Xia E, Xiao Y, Li TC, Huang X, Liu Y. Management of false passage created during hysteroscopic adhesiolysis for Asherman's syndrome. Journal of Obstetrics and Gynaecology. 2016;**36**(1):87-92

[24] Darwish AM, Ahmad AM, Mohammad AM. Cervical priming prior to operative hysteroscopy: A randomized comparison of laminaria versus misoprostol. Human Reproduction. 2004;**19**(10):2391-2394

[25] Casadei L, Piccolo E, Manicuti C, Cardinale S, Collamarini M, Piccione E. Role of vaginal estradiol pretreatment combined with vaginal misoprostol for cervical ripening before operative hysteroscopy in postmenopausal women. Obstetrics & Gynecology Science. 2016;**59**(3):220-226

[26] Skopec GS. A review of medical and surgical techniques for overcoming cervical stenosis. Proceedings in Obstetrics and Gynecology. 2018;**8**(1):1-7

[27] Salari BW, Bhagavath B, Galloway ML, Findley AD, Yaklic JL, Lindheim SR. Hysteroscopic morcellator to overcome cervical stenosis. Fertility and Sterility. 2016;**106**(6):e12-e13

[28] Kresowik JD, Syrop CH, Van Voorhis BJ, Ryan GL. Ultrasound is the optimal choice for guidance in difficult hysteroscopy. Ultrasound in Obstetrics & Gynecology. 2012;**39**(6):715-718

[29] Christianson MS, Barker MA, Lindheim SR. Overcoming the challenging cervix: Techniques to access the uterine cavity. Journal of Lower Genital Tract Disease. 2008;**12**(1):24-31

[30] Aas-Eng MK, Langebrekke A, Hudelist G. Complications in operative hysteroscopy–is prevention possible? Acta Obstetricia et Gynecologica Scandinavica. 2017;**96**(12):1399-1403

[31] Bradley LD. Complications in hysteroscopy: Prevention, treatment and legal risk. Current Opinion in Obstetrics & Gynecology. 2002;**14**(4):409-415

[32] Paschopoulos M, Polyzos NP, Lavasidis LG, Vrekoussis T, Dalkalitsis N, Paraskevaidis E. Safety issues of hysteroscopic surgery. Annals of the New York Academy of Sciences. 2006;**1092**:229-234

[33] Macdonald R. Endometrial ablation: A safe procedure. Gynaecological Endoscopy. 1992;**1**:7-9

[34] MacLean-Fraser E, Penava D, Vilos GA. Perioperative complication rates of primary and repeat hysteroscopic endometrial ablations. The Journal of the American Association of Gynecologic Laparoscopists. 2002;**9**(2):175-177

[35] Shakir F, Diab Y. The perforated uterus. The Obstetrician & Gynaecologist. 2013;**15**(4):256-261

[36] Hulka JF, Peterson HB, Phillips JM, Surrey MW. Operative hysteroscopy. American Association of Gynecologic Laparoscopists 1991 membership survey. The Journal of Reproductive Medicine. 1993;**38**(8):572-573

[37] Agostini A, Cravello L, Desbrière R, Maisonneuve AS, Roger V, Blanc B. Hemorrhage risk during operative hysteroscopy. Acta Obstetricia et Gynecologica Scandinavica. 2002;**81**(9):878-881

[38] Loffer FD. Removing intrauterine lesions: Myomectomy and polypectomy. In: Bibier EJ, Loffer FD. editors. Hysteroscopy, Resectoscopy and Endometrial Ablation(1st ed.). New York: CRC Press; 2003. pp. 149-166

[39] Fonseca MDF, Andrade Junior CM, Nogueira EDA, Sessa FV, Crispi CP. Predictors of fluid intravasation during operative hysteroscopy: A preplanned prospective observational study with 200 cases. Revista Brasileira de Ginecologia e Obstetrícia. 2015;**37**:24-29

[40] Phillips DR, Nathanson HG, Milim SJ, Haselkorn JS, Khapra A, Ross PL. The effect of dilute vasopressin solution on blood loss during operative hysteroscopy: A randomized controlled trial. Obstetrics & Gynecology. 1996;**88**(5):761-766

[41] Hobo R, Netsu S, Koyasu Y, Tsutsumi O. Bradycardia and cardiac arrest caused by intramyometrial injection of vasopressin during a laparoscopically assisted myomectomy. Obstetrics & Gynecology. 2009;**113**(2):484-486

[42] Park KS, Yoo KY. Role of vasopressin in current anesthetic practice. Korean Journal of Anesthesiology. 2017;**70**(3):245-257

[43] Goldrath MH. Uterine tamponade for the control of acute uterine bleeding. American Journal of Obstetrics and Gynecology. 1983;**147**(8):869-872

[44] Mushambi MC, Williamson K. Anaesthetic considerations for hysteroscopic surgery. Best practice & research. Clinical Anaesthesiology. 2002;**16**(1):35-52

[45] Umranikar S, Clark TJ, Saridogan E, Miligkos D, Arambage K, Torbe E, et al. BSGE/ESGE guideline on management of fluid distension media in operative hysteroscopy. Gynecological Surgery. 2016;**13**(4):289-303

[46] Worldwide AAMIG. AAGL practice report: Practice guidelines for the management of hysteroscopic distending media:(replaces hysteroscopic fluid monitoring guidelines. J Am Assoc Gynecol Laparosc. 2000; 7: 167-168.). Journal of Minimally Invasive Gynecology. 2013;**20**(2):137-148

[47] Witz CA, Silverberg KM, Burns WN, Schenken RS, Olive DL. Complications associated with the absorption of hysteroscopic fluid media. Fertility and Sterility. 1993;**60**(5):745-756

[48] Baggish MS, Brill AI, Rosenweig B, Barbot JE, Indman PD. Fatal acute glycine and sorbitol toxicity during operative hysteroscopy. Journal of Gynecologic Surgery. 1993;**9**(3):137-143

[49] Ayus JC, Wheeler JM, Arieff AI. Postoperative hyponatremic

encephalopathy in menstruant women. Annals of Internal Medicine. 1992;**117**(11):891-897

[50] Karci A, Erkin Y. Transient blindness following hysteroscopy. Journal of International Medical Research. 2003;**31**(2):152-155

[51] Shirk GJ, Gimpelson RJ. Control of intrauterine fluid pressure during opermunroative hysteroscopy. The Journal of the American Association of Gynecologic Laparoscopists. 1994;**1**(3):229-233

[52] Varol N, Maher P, Vancaillie T, Cooper M, Carter J, Kwok A, et al. A literature review and update on the prevention and management of fluid overload in endometrial resection and hysteroscopic surgery. Gynaecological Endoscopy. 2002;**11**(1):19-26

[53] Munro MG. Complications of hysteroscopic and uterine resectoscopic surgery. Obstetrics and Gynecology Clinics of North America. 2010;**37**(3):399-425

[54] Irvin W, Andersen W, Taylor P, Rice L. Minimizing the risk of neurologic injury in gynecologic surgery. Obstetrics and Gynecology. 2004;**103**(2):374-382

[55] Kuponiyi O, Alleemudder DI, Latunde-Dada A, Eedarapalli P. Nerve injuries associated with gynaecological surgery. The Obstetrician & Gynaecologist. 2014;**16**(1):29-36

[56] Bradshaw AD, Advincula AP. Postoperative neuropathy in gynecologic surgery. Obstetrics and Gynecology Clinics of North America. 2010;**37**(3):451-459

[57] Batres F, Barclay DL. Sciatic nerve injury during gynecologic procedures using the lithotomy position. Obstetrics and Gynecology. 1983;**62** (3 Suppl):92s-94s

[58] Abdalmageed OS, Bedaiwy MA, Falcone T. Nerve injuries in gynecologic laparoscopy. Journal of Minimally Invasive Gynecology. 2017;**24**(1):16-27

[59] Sobolewski B, Doman P, Stetkiewicz T, Oszukowski P, Woźniak P. The toxic impact of local anaesthetics in menopausal women: Causes, prevention and treatment after local anaesthetic overdose. Local anaesthetic systemic toxicity syndrome. Menopause Review/Przegląd Menopauzalny. 2015;**14**(1):65-70

[60] Riff C, Le Caloch A, Dupouey J, Allanioux L, Leone M, Blin O, et al. Local anesthetic plasma concentrations as a valuable tool to confirm the diagnosis of local anesthetic systemic toxicity? A report of 10 years of experience. Pharmaceutics. 2022;**14**(4):708

[61] El-Boghdadly K, Pawa A, Chin KJ. Local anesthetic systemic toxicity: Current perspectives. Local and Regional Anesthesia. 2018;**11**:35

[62] Ciechanowicz S, Patil V. Lipid emulsion for local anesthetic systemic toxicity. Anesthesiology research and practice. 2012;**2012**:131784

[63] Roman RA, Roberts CC, Booth R, Lindheim SR. Crisis Management in the Office Setting. In: Reproductive Surgery. Cham: Springer; 2022. pp. 269-278

[64] Gupta N, Gupta A. Commentary: Venous air embolism during hysteroscopy: A stitch in time saves nine! Journal of Anaesthesiology, Clinical Pharmacology. 2019;**35**(3):417

[65] Groenman FA, Peters LW, Rademaker BM, Bakkum EA. Embolism of air and gas in hysteroscopic

procedures: Pathophysiology and implication for daily practice. Journal of Minimally Invasive Gynecology. 2008;**15**(2):241-247

[66] Chen M, Zhao M, Yang Y, Tang H, Qin Z, Liu J, et al. Air embolism: A severe complication of Hysteroscopic surgery. Journal of Gynecology and Obstetrics. 2022;**10**(4):171-175

[67] Lowenwirt IP, Chi DS, Handwerker SM. Nonfatal venous air embolism during cesarean section: A case report and review of the literature. Obstetrical & Gynecological Survey. 1994;**49**(1):72-76

[68] Dyrbye BA, Overdijk LE, van Kesteren PJ, de Haan P, Riezebos RK, Bakkum EA, et al. Gas embolism during hysteroscopic surgery using bipolar or monopolar diathermia: A randomized controlled trial. American Journal of Obstetrics and Gynecology. 2012;**207**(4):271-2e1

[69] Brull SJ, Prielipp RC. Vascular air embolism: A silent hazard to patient safety. Journal of Critical Care. 2017;**42**:255-263

[70] Storm BS, Andreasen S, Hovland A, Nielsen EW. Gas embolism during hysteroscopic surgery?: Three cases and a literature review. A&A Practice. 2017;**9**(5):140-143

[71] Rubal BJ, Leon A, Meyers BL, Bell CM. The 'mill-wheel' murmur and computed tomography of intracardiac air emboli. Journal of the American Association for Laboratory Animal Science: JAALAS. 2009;**48**(3):300-302

[72] McCarthy CJ, Behravesh S, Naidu SG, Oklu R. Air embolism: Practical tips for prevention and treatment. Journal of Clinical Medicine. 2016;**5**(11):93

[73] Ratner RT, Tsaltas J, Vollenhoven B. Hysteroscopy and the risk of gas embolism: A review. Journal of Endometriosis and Pelvic Pain Disorders. 2020;**12**(1):51-55

[74] Agostini A, Cravello L, Shojai R, Ronda I, Roger V, Blanc B. Postoperative infection and surgical hysteroscopy. Fertility and Sterility. 2002;**77**(4):766-768

[75] Kasius JC, Broekmans FJ, Fauser BC, Devroey P, Fatemi HM. Antibiotic prophylaxis for hysteroscopy evaluation of the uterine cavity. Fertility and Sterility. 2011;**95**(2):792-794

[76] Muzii L, Di Donato V, Boni T, Gaglione R, Marana R, Mazzon I, et al. Antibiotics prophylaxis for operative hysteroscopy. Reproductive sciences (Thousand Oaks, Calif.). 2017;**24**(4): 534-538

[77] Nappi L, Di Spiezio Sardo A, Spinelli M, Guida M, Mencaglia L, Greco P, et al. A multicenter, double-blind, randomized, placebo-controlled study to assess whether antibiotic administration should be recommended during office operative hysteroscopy. Reproductive sciences (Thousand Oaks, Calif.). 2013;**20**(7):755-761

[78] Price TM, Harris JB. Fulminant hepatic failure due to herpes simplex after hysteroscopy. Obstetrics & Gynecology. 2001;**98**(5):954-956

[79] Hill DJ. Hematometra-a complication of endometrial ablation/resection. The Journal of the American Association of Gynecologic Laparoscopists. 1994;**1**(4, Part 2):S14-S14

[80] Hubert SR, Marcus PS, Rothenberg JM, Schilder JM, Hurd WW. Hematometra after thermal balloon endometrial ablation in a patient with cervical incompetence. Journal of Laparoendoscopic & Advanced Surgical Techniques. 2001;**11**(5):311-313

[81] McCausland AM, McCausland VM. Long-term complications of endometrial ablation: Cause, diagnosis, treatment, and prevention. Journal of Minimally Invasive Gynecology. 2007;**14**(4):399-406

[82] McCausland AM, McCausland VM. Long-term complications of minimally invasive endometrial ablation devices. Journal of Gynecologic Surgery. 2010;**26**(2):133-149

[83] Hill D. Complications of operative hysteroscopy. Gynecology Endoscopy. 1992;**1**:7

[84] Townsend DE, McCausland V, McCausland A, Fields G, Kauffman K. s rPost-ablation-tubal sterilization syndrome. Obstetrics and Gynecology. 1993;**82**(3):422-424

[85] Webb JC, Bush MR, Wood MD, Park GS. Hematosalpinx with pelvic pain after endometrial ablation confirms the postablation-tubal sterilization syndrome. The Journal of the American Association of Gynecologic Laparoscopists. 1996;**3**(3):419-421

[86] McCausland AM, McCausland VM. Frequency of symptomatic cornual hematometra and postablation tubal sterilization syndrome after total rollerball endometrial ablation: A 10-year follow-up. American Journal of Obstetrics and Gynecology. 2002;**186**(6):1274-1283

[87] Cooper JM, Brady RM. Late complications of operative hysteroscopy. Obstetrics and Gynecology Clinics of North America. 2000;**27**(2):367-374

[88] Leung PL, Yuen PM. Postablation–tubal sterilization syndrome following thermal balloon endometrial ablation. Acta Obstetricia et Gynecologica Scandinavica. 2006;**85**(4):504-505

[89] Tam T, Elgar C, Jirschele K, Lombard E. Post-ablation tubal sterilization syndrome following NovaSure endometrial ablation: Two case reports. Gynecological Surgery. 2012;**9**(4):449-452

[90] Taskin O, Sadik S, Onoglu A, Gokdeniz R, Erturan E, Burak F, et al. Role of endometrial suppression on the frequency of intrauterine adhesions after resectoscopic surgery. The Journal of the American Association of Gynecologic Laparoscopists. 2000;**7**(3):351-354

[91] Malhotra N, Okohue JE. Adhesions and Asherman. In: Atlas of Hysteroscopy. Cham: Springer; 2020. pp. 73-82

[92] Conforti A, Alviggi C, Mollo A, De Placido G, Magos A. The management of Asherman syndrome: A review of literature. Reproductive Biology and Endocrinology. 2013;**11**(1):1-11

[93] Warembourg S, Huberlant S, Garric X, Leprince S, de Tayrac R, Letouzey V. Prévention et traitement des synéchies endo-utérines : revue de la littérature. Journal de Gynécologie Obstétrique et Biologie de la Reproduction. 2015;**44**(4):366-379

[94] Nelson LD, Grobman WA. Obstetric morbidity associated with amniotic sheets. Ultrasound in Obstetrics & Gynecology. 2010;**36**:324-327

[95] Zikopoulos KA, Kolibianakis EM, Platteau P, De Munck L, Tournaye H, Devroey P, et al. Live delivery rates in subfertile women with Asherman's syndrome after hysteroscopic adhesiolysis using the resectoscope or the Versapoint system. Reproductive Biomedicine Online. 2004;**8**(6):720-725

[96] Fedele L, Vercellini P, Viezzoli T, Ricciardiello O, Zamberletti D. Intrauterine adhesions: Current diagnostic and therapeutic trends. Acta Europaea Fertilitatis. 1986;**17**(1):31-37

[97] Guo EJ, Chung JPW, Poon LCY, Li TC. Reproductive outcomes after surgical treatment of asherman syndrome: A systematic review. Best Practice & Research Clinical Obstetrics & Gynaecology. 2019;**59**:98-114

[98] Duffy S, Reid PC, Sharp F. In-vivo studies of uterine electrosurgery. BJOG: An International Journal of Obstetrics & Gynaecology. 1992;**99**:579-582

[99] Sebbag L, Even M, Fay S, Naoura I, Revaux A, Carbonnel M, et al. Early second-look hysteroscopy: Prevention and treatment of intrauterine post-surgical adhesions. Frontiers in Surgery. 2019;**6**:50

[100] Tonguc EA, Var T, Yilmaz N, Batioglu S. Intrauterine device or estrogen treatment after hysteroscopic uterine septum resection. International Journal of Gynecology & Obstetrics. 2010;**109**(3):226-229

[101] Lin X, Wei M, Li TC, Huang Q, Huang D, Zhou F, et al. A comparison of intrauterine balloon, intrauterine contraceptive device and hyaluronic acid gel in the prevention of adhesion reformation following hysteroscopic surgery for Asherman syndrome: A cohort study. European Journal of Obstetrics & Gynecology and Reproductive Biology. 2013;**170**(2):512-516

[102] Orhue AA, Aziken ME, Igbefoh JO. A comparison of two adjunctive treatments for intrauterine adhesions following lysis. International Journal of Gynaecology and Obstetrics: The Official Organ of the International Federation of Gynaecology and Obstetrics. 2003;**82**(1):49-56

[103] Guida M. Effectiveness of auto-crosslinked hyaluronic acid gel in the prevention of intrauterine adhesions after hysteroscopic surgery: A prospective, randomized, controlled study. Human Reproduction. 2004;**19**(6): 1461-1464

[104] Bosteels J, Weyers S, Mol BW, D'Hooghe T. Anti-adhesion barrier gels following operative hysteroscopy for treating female infertility: A systematic review and meta-analysis. Gynecological Surgery. 2014;**11**(2):113-127

[105] Römer T, Schmidt T, Foth D. Pre- and postoperative hormonal treatment in patients with hysteroscopic surgery. Contributions to Gynecology and Obstetrics. 2000;**20**:1-12

[106] Nagori CB, Panchal SY, Patel H. Endometrial regeneration using autologous adult stem cells followed by conception by in vitro fertilization in a patient of severe Asherman's syndrome. Journal of Human Reproductive Sciences. 2011;**4**(1):43

[107] Gimpelson RJ. Ten-year literature review of global endometrial ablation with the NovaSure® device. International Journal of Women's Health. 2014;**6**:269-280. DOI: 10.2147/IJWH.S56364

[108] Wortman M. Endometrial ablation: Past, present, and future part II. Surgical Technology International. 2018;**33**:161-177

[109] Gervaise A, de Tayrac R, Fernandez H. Contraceptive information after endometrial ablation. Fertility and Sterility. 2005;**84**(6):1746-1747

[110] Kohn JR, Shamshirsaz AA, Popek E, Guan X, Belfort MA, Fox KA. Pregnancy after endometrial ablation: A systematic review. BJOG: An International Journal of Obstetrics & Gynaecology. 2018;**125**(1):43-53

[111] Sharp HT. Endometrial ablation: Postoperative complications. American Journal of Obstetrics and Gynecology. 2012;**207**(4):242-247

[112] Yin CS. Pregnancy after hysteroscopic endometrial ablation without endometrial preparation: A report of five cases and a literature review. Taiwanese Journal of Obstetrics and Gynecology. 2010;**49**(3):311-319

[113] Giarenis I, Shenoy J, Morris E. Cervical ectopic pregnancy after endometrial ablation: A case report. Archives of Gynecology and Obstetrics. 2008;**277**(6):567-569

[114] Lo JS, Pickersgill A. Pregnancy after endometrial ablation: English literature review and case report. Journal of Minimally Invasive Gynecology. 2006;**13**(2):88-91

[115] Conturso R, Redaelli L, Pasini A, Tenore A. Spontaneous uterine rupture with amniotic sac protrusion at 28 weeks subsequent to previous hysteroscopic metroplasty. European Journal of Obstetrics, Gynecology, and Reproductive Biology. 2003;**107**:98-100

[116] Howe RS. Third-trimester uterine rupture following hysteron scopic uterine perforation. Part 2. Obstetrics and Gynecology. 1993;**81**(5):827

[117] Yaron Y, Shenhav M, Jaffa AJ, Lessing JB, Peyser MR. Uterine rupture at 33 weeks' gestation subsequent to hysteroscopic uterine perforation. American Journal of Obstetrics and Gynecology. 1994;**170**(3):786-787

[118] Lobaugh ML, Bammel BM, Duke D, et al. Uterine rupture during pregnancy in a patient with a history of hysteroscopic uterine perforation. American Journal of Obstetrics and Gynecology. 1994;**83**:838-840

[119] Angell NF, Domingo JT, Siddiqi N. Uterine rupture at term after uncomplicated hysteroscopic metroplasty. Obstetrics & Gynecology. 2002;**100**(5):1098-1099

[120] Deaton IL, Maier D, Andreoli J. Spontaneous uterine rupture during pregnancy after treatment of Asherman's syndrome. American Journal of Obstetrics and Gynecology. 1989;**160**:1053-1054

[121] Friedman A, DeFazio J, DeCherney A. Severe obstetrical complications after aggressive treatment of Asherman syndrome. Obstetrics and Gynecology. 1986;**67**:864-867

[122] Ergenoglu M, Yeniel AO, Yıldırım N, Akdemir A, Yucebilgin S. Recurrent uterine rupture after hysteroscopic resection of the uterine septum. International Journal of Surgery Case Reports. 2013;**4**:182-184

[123] Abbas A, Irvine LM. Uterine rupture during labour after hysteroscopic myomectomy. Gynaecological Endoscopy. 1997;**6**(4):245-246

[124] Tinelli A, Kosmas IP, Carugno JT, Carp H, Malvasi A, Cohen SB, et al. Uterine rupture during pregnancy: The URIDA (uterine rupture international data acquisition) study. International Journal of Gynecology & Obstetrics. 2022;**157**(1):76-84

[125] Sentilhes L, Sergent F, Roman H, Verspyck E, Marpeau L. Late complications of operative hysteroscopy: Predicting patients at risk of uterine rupture during subsequent pregnancy. European Journal of Obstetrics & Gynecology and Reproductive Biology. 2005;**120**(2):134-138

[126] Gürgan T, Yarali H, Urman B, Dagli V, Dogan L. Uterine rupture following hysteroscopic lysis of synechiae due to tuberculosis and uterine perforation. Human Reproduction (Oxford, England). 1996;**11**(2):291-293